"*The Adventures of Canc[er Bitch is...]* and honest. Wisenberg ha[s...] she is willing to tell all [...] information as well as a very smart, funny read from an excellent writer."
— **Audrey Niffenegger, author of *The Time Traveler's Wife***

"Read *The Adventures of Cancer Bitch* to meet a smart, funny, big-hearted woman who questions everything from her own mortality to career envy to why nobody thinks the particulars of hair-loss are as fascinating a subject for extended dinner-party conversation as she does. Along the way, Wisenberg makes you proud to think that you, too, might possibly be a cancer bitch."
— **Ruth Pennebaker, author of *Women on the Verge of a Nervous Breakthrough***

"Dealing with cancer is a bitch—and the complexity of writing about it in a way that reflects on the very process of writing is really, really hard. Sandi Wisenberg's account of her diagnosis, treatment, and lives, before and after, forces her and us into our collective history. Having written well about the Holocaust, as she has admirably done, suddenly places her account of her illness into a new re-reading of the past, the present, and the future. Brilliant written; extraordinarily moving."
— **Sander L. Gilman, author of *Difference and Pathology***

"Frank, funny, fierce, and at times devastating, *Cancer Bitch* is a rare achievement. S. L. Wisenberg has written a book of tremendous value for anyone who has ever had cancer or anyone who has ever worried about getting it; in short, everyone."
— **Rachel Schukert, writer, producer, *The Baby-Sitters Club* and *GLOW***

"Best book for someone who likes the idea of the Oprah Book Club but thinks they're too cool....[It] manages to dodge much of the maudlin retrospectivity of crisis or illness memoirs. Instead, the reader gets a sense of the immediate reactions and turbulent emotions experienced by a patient as news and developments filter down from doctors."
— ***Time Out* Chicago**

"...like the best of the savage memoirs, it's doused in hope, and as readers, we share a most important reward in the end: life."
— ***Newcity***

"...defiant, combative, uses humor strategically." Wisenberg uses "cancer as a subversive muse."
— **Mary K. DeShazer, author of *Mammographies: The Cultural Discourses of Breast Cancer***

It's "damned funny…But….she settles into a register of high seriousness without a trace of self importance."
— *Bookslut*

"She's not a bitch but a woman who has faced a life-threatening illness with defiance and courage, and who, even when she's raging or struggling against it can look outside herself and be a part of the world around her."
— *Chicago Jewish Star*

"As a reader, it is easy to feel her stress and sympathize as if you are on the sofa next to her as she wallows in her pain. This pain does not make Wisenberg bitchy; on the contrary, it reveals her true character questioning the world around her and why the commodified pink ribbons have become a 'catch-all' for the destructive disease we all encounter at some point in our lives."
— *Feminist Review*

"*The Adventures of Cancer Bitch* is among the most Jewish of the recent memoirs. It is also among the most poetic."
— *Jewish Woman* **magazine**

"She demonstrates her talents easily…." The book "reads like someone who has thrown herself open to the experience, emotionally and intellectually buffeted by the currents, recording everything just as it washes over her."
— **Being Cancer Network**

"…a must-read for anyone you think is tough enough to take it. Wry, refreshingly (and some times brutally) honest and clinically graphic, her first-person account of dealing with breast cancer has gems of experience and insight."
— *Herizons* **Magazine**

The Adventures of Cancer Bitch

The Adventures of Cancer Bitch

S.L. Wisenberg

Tortoise Books

Chicago

SECOND EDITION, OCTOBER, 2024

Copyright © 2024 by Sandi Wisenberg

All rights reserved under International and Pan-American Copyright Convention
Published in the United States by Tortoise Books

www.tortoisebooks.com

ISBN-13: 978-1948954938

This book is a chronicle and a memoir, and is drawn from the author's experiences and recollections. Dialogue ranges from precise re-creation to approximate. To protect privacy, names and identifying details have either been omitted or changed.

Front Cover: Based on Shutterstock image 2265100467. Copyright ©2024 by Tortoise Books. Original artwork by Gerald Brennan.

Tortoise Books Logo Copyright ©2024 by Tortoise Books. Original artwork by Rachele O'Hare.

January 16. Cells Gone Wild

It begins with a whiff of criminality: a *suspicious* place on a routine mammogram. Something fishy. On the film, a dark circle that doesn't belong there. *There* being my body. The body that has, perhaps, gone wild. On the cellular level. Cancer is overproduction, the assembly belt gone haywire, the sorcerer's broom wheeling out of control when the apprentice thinks he knows enough. Too much too much too many. The experts examine and pick and remain close-lipped. It could be something. Or nothing. But they say *or nothing* as an afterthought. Because they know it's cancer but they can't say it yet because Pathology hasn't said so. And then Pathology says so. And then the radiology fellow says: It's positive. The surgeon says, It's in three places, not one, and we'll have to take off the whole breast, we can't conserve it.

It sounds like it happens fast but it doesn't. There is much waiting, in the hospital in a pale blue gown that's both too loose and too tight with those little blue ties that never match up. There are phone calls. The whole thing—is a relief in a way. Because with every mammogram I've ever had, I've gone through cancer scenarios in my head: all the way to whether I'll have an obituary in the *Chicago Tribune* written by a staff writer (a news obituary) or whether my husband Linc will have to pay for a death notice. I wonder whether he'll sit *shiva* (Of course not) or if my mother will (Yes, of course). And I worry about my papers. My words—my six tall file cabinets filled with finished and unfinished manuscripts, letters from the days when people wrote letters, accounts of dreams from the early 1980s. Where will they go? No archivist has ever come calling, asking for everything. Or anything.

I'm wondering about the papers but I'm really wondering about my self. If it's cancer and if I die of it, my body will go to science. And then I will be gone from this earth.

January 16. Hematology

The day I went for the follow-up mammogram I also had an appointment with a hematologist because I have a high platelet count—high enough to be monitored but not to require intervention. The official name is essential thrombocythemia. Before the doctor came in, a fourth-year medical student interviewed me to practice his skills. He was nervous and hadn't read my chart. I was telling him about my long menstrual periods, which supposedly aren't related to the low amount of iron in my blood, according to doctors, but I think really are. I said, in explanation, I have fibroids. Oh, he said, I'm one of three boys. Pause. He mumbled: What did you say? I pretended I didn't hear him, but for a moment imagined the spectre of five sons, imagined them around me in the patient room. I explained: Fibroids. Uterine fibroids.

January 24. How NOT to Tell Your Class About Your Breast Cancer

1. Be grateful that during class you don't think about your cancer, except during free-writing, when they're making lists that begin with Because, using as a model a poem by Susan Donnelly called "Why I Can't." The title of your list is: *Why I Don't Trust Doctors Who Are Very Good-looking.*

2. Tell them as soon as you know, on the day you get your terse diagnosis from Cold Blonde, the good-looking radiology fellow at the hospital. Don't wait until you have concrete information that your students will need, such as dates of classes you will miss.

3. Wait until five minutes before class ends. While they are standing with their coats on, say that you have something to tell them. That you have breast cancer. Expect your voice to be calm. It will not be. It will break. You will be in danger of crying. Tell them you will find substitutes for any classes you'll miss. Tell them you're going to talk to a surgeon the next day, but be unable to continue, leaving them stunned. Then exit.

4. On the way home, think about how irresponsible you were.

5. At home, send an e-mail to all of them, telling them you're sorry if you freaked them out. Become paranoid when only one of them replies.

6. Have a friend tell you that it's all about what you need, so whatever you needed to do was OK. Know that she's wrong. Your job, in a way, is to protect your students from your own *mishegoss*.

7. Post this on the class's website and see what happens.

January 25. Surgeon

The surgeon is warm but businesslike, a nice combination. She says the cancer is probably stage 2, because the mass is probably more than 5 cm. But I thought it was 2 cm. She explains that now they're thinking of the three places as one big place. Surgery would be in two to three weeks. Without reconstruction, the hospital stay would be one to two days. With, four to five.

I tell her I don't want reconstruction. I've thought about it—because I've had two breast biopsies, the first more than twenty years ago; because I know women who've had breast cancer; because I know that it's an epidemic; because I've seen that poster of Deena Metzger naked with a tattoo over her mastectomy scar; I've imagined how I would react to losing a breast. (But not losing two, that's too much to take on.) I've thought that I would be defiantly one-breasted. My breasts are small, too small for cleavage, growing from A to B only fairly recently as I've gained some weight. I like them small. They make me look thinner and don't get in my way. The only reason for me to wear a bra is to provide a little uplift and to cover my nipples. They stick out all the time, like erasers on a pencil.

The surgeon says I should talk to the plastic surgeon anyway, just to see what my options are. And then suddenly, I, who'd imagined myself a fierce, one-breasted Amazon, find myself thinking: I would love to have reconstruction.

January 27. Tank Top

    Wendy has graciously offered to talk to me about reconstruction after her mastectomy. She greets me at her suburban door in a red tank top with black bra straps showing. The top is tucked into white pants. In the midst of winter she's dressing for summer. Indicating her clothes, she says, I'm not wearing this just for you. Her treatments have zapped her into instant menopause and she's suffering from hot flashes. But why shouldn't she wear her tank top? She looks fine in it. And later, when she shows me both breasts, I see that they're almost identical, except for the long scar on top across one of them. She lets me push a little on the new breast so I can tell that it's soft. She has silicone implants and praises her plastic surgeon to the skies: he loves women's breasts, she says. She also recommends her breast surgeon. All was done at what I'll call Plain Hospital, though she tells me you can pick and choose your surgeons and oncologists and pathologists, they can be at different institutions. She sent her slides to a certain pathologist in Tennessee who she says is world-famous. The idea of doing that seems daunting, but why not? She says that my hospital—which I call Fancy, because the first floor looks like a hotel lobby—misread her pathology report.
    I've never before touched another woman's breasts. My idea of teenage-hood and life was much influenced by *The Diary of a Young Girl* (Anne Frank), read at a very early age. I remember she talked about asking a friend if she could touch her breasts. Her friend said no. I thought it must be a normal thing to ask another girl. But I never did.

January 27. I Love Pink M&M's®

I love pink M&M's®. I eat them every day. That's all I eat. If I eat enough of them my cancer will go away. Won't it? Isn't that what they promise? In the USA we like our news and health and our donations sugar-coated. If I eat M&M's® and if I go on the Avon Walk (Do I get a free Avon makeover before setting out; all those cameras, you see; I must look my best; it's important to look my best; that's why we wear pink ribbons in our hair and—oops—some of us don't have hair; then around our necks?) and if I sell Pink Ribbon Cupcakes and Support the Cause Brownies (*Great for a bake sale or afternoon tea*, the Pink Ribbon folks suggest.) then I will be in the pink. The ingredients for Support the Cause Brownies will make me healthy. If not, why would they be named after Susan G. Komen, who has a whole breast cancer foundation named after her? Oops—she's dead. She died of breast cancer. Maybe she died from eating these brownies. But how could that be? They're made with M&M's® Milk Chocolate Candies Help Fight Breast Cancer, mixed with Snickers, and brownie mix (any brand—quick, here's an opportunity for another multinational corporation to hop on the Pink bandwagon) and a can of (your brand name here) chocolate frosting. What could be more natural for us girls? We're made of sugar and spice. Even our out-of-control cancer cells are nice. Because they're pink, like us. Aren't they? Remember to follow the recipe. We have to learn to follow recipes to be good cancer patients. And don't forget the final decorations. Decorations are important. *Make a continuous ring of M&M's® Brand Milk Chocolate Candies Help Fight Breast Cancer around the bottom of the brownies.* Celebrate!

◆ ◆ ◆

Or instead of baking, you could read a book, like *Pink Ribbons, Inc: Breast Cancer and the Politics of Philanthropy* by Samantha King, which says:

> *As the Komen Foundation and its corporate sponsors continue to pump money into a research and education agenda that centers on uncritically promoting mammography, encouraging the use of pharmaceuticals to 'prevent' breast cancer, and avoiding any consideration of environmental links to the disease it becomes less clear whether they are not actually doing more harm than good....*

January 31. Plastic Surgeon

I had an appointment with a plastic surgeon Wednesday afternoon at Fancy Hospital. He showed me before and after photos of patients. He said that reconstructed breasts are high and round and don't look exactly like breasts. Once he said that, I thought, Hey, they look like orange halves. He recommended saline implants for me, even though their infection rate is one in twenty. That's mostly for smokers and D-sizes, he said. As he left the examining room he said I needed to have my picture taken (meaning pictures of my breasts) so that he could remember me. *Les seins, ce sont moi.*

♦ ♦ ♦

Just a few minutes ago my computer told me that Molly Ivins is dead, at sixty-two. Of breast cancer. She had Inflammatory Breast Cancer, which is not what I have. (Whew. Knowing it's selfish to be relieved.) IBC is less common than what I have, and has very different symptoms. It is amazing that she wrote almost up until the very end, which is what I plan to do.

More January 31. Free Dinners

Linc has noticed that everyone wanted to give us dinner. Our second one was with our neighbor Anand. He and his wife are what the French call *les voisins de palier*, meaning neighbors on the same floor. I suppose there were more apartment buildings earlier on in France than, say, England, and thus the phrase was invented. I don't know if there are equivalents in other languages spoken in densely-populated cities. We ate at the Neighborhood Veggie Place Where Not Enough is Organic. We got to talking about nipples. I said mine had to be removed in the mastectomy, because there might be disease in it. Linc said it was preserved, that he was paying attention to that part of the surgeon's talk. What did he think, it can be moved around like a maraschino cherry on a sundae? (I looked it up later. It can be cut and replaced in some surgeries, but not at Fancy Hospital, according to the pink handbook the hospital gave me. The handbook is the size of the original *Our Bodies, Our Selves*, and I pasted a medusa over the pink rose on the cover.) We were also talking about donating bone marrow for some reason. Anand has plans to see if he's a match for someone who needs a donor. Linc said he had been planning to donate marrow or plasma to a woman in his office, but... she died. Oh, I said, pretty sure I knew who he was talking about, of breast cancer? Yes. For some reason I started laughing. Then I told Anand how my friend Peggy had offered to loan me books, one of which is *The Cancer Journals* by Audre Lorde, who died of breast cancer. I don't want books by people who died of it.

I also told Peggy a few days before how I was inwardly scoffing about someone who recommended Plain Hospital, because she'd gotten a biopsy there. Only a biopsy? That's *bupkes*. I said it's the way Holocaust survivors have a hierarchy. The ones who survived Auschwitz look down on the ones who were only in concentration camps (rather than extermination camps), and the people who were in the concentration camps look down on the ones who were only in labor camps, and those people look down on the ones who spent the war in hiding. So the friend who had the biopsy, I said, it was like she was hiding in a barn the whole time. A nice barn, out of the way of soldiers and hostile peasants.

And the ones who died? Peggy asked. Where would they fit in?

February 3. Whodunit: Two Household Mysteries

1. The plumber came to figure out why water leaked downstairs when I took a long shower. After running the water and going downstairs and back, he couldn't figure it out, because of course it didn't leak when he was here. It could be that the water had splashed on the tile and there was a hole in the grout.

2. I have breast cancer and no one knows where it came from. Pollution and pesticides? What about all the other people who didn't get it and live in the same environment? Additives in cosmetics and creams? See previous. Genes? No first-degree relatives—mother, grandmothers, sister—have had it. No pregnancies? That's a risk factor.

I don't know much about the history of breast cancer. I know that the first patient described (as a young woman) in Freud and Breuer's *Case Studies on Hysteria* lived into her seventies and died of breast cancer, in 1936. No, wait, that was intestinal. There must be histories of it in ancient Egypt, Rome, etc. Nothing in the Bible as far as I know. (Pause for Google search.) I find a recent book, *Bathsheba's Breast: Women, Cancer, and History*, by James S. Olson. From the book description: *A horror known to every culture in every age, breast cancer has been responsible for the deaths of 25 million women throughout history. An Egyptian physician writing 3,500 years ago concluded that there was no treatment for the disease.*

More February 3. Teapot / *Société Anonyme*

Our third free meal was with our good friends Posey and Marv. They have Italian ceramic dinnerware, as we do, but in a different pattern. They have mostly Raffaellesco, with a yellow dragon in the middle, and we have a mix of Veccio Deruta and Arabesco. Last year my friend Garnett gave me a Raffaellesco teapot. At dinner when Posey and Marv were in the other room, I whispered to Linc that when I'm gone he should give them my teapot. Gone, as in dead.

Do I really think I will die soon, before Linc, before Posey and Marv (who are about fifteen years older than I am), meaning, that I will die from this? No one dies from breast cancer, as long as it stays in the breast; you die from the spread of the breast cancer cells to other parts of your body. There's no sign—yet—that it's spread. I've thought about death a lot, from an early age. I've had asthma since babyhood; if you have trouble breathing, you're bound to imagine what it would like to stop breathing for good. I read Anne Frank's diary when I was seven or eight, and I would picture the Nazis coming to get us. My sister and I would pretend that we were teachers or secretaries, like our other friends did, but we also would sit hunched and whispering in our pink walk-in closets in Texas and pretend we were in hiding from the Nazis.

I imagined that I would go like that (snap o' fingers) if I were taken to a concentration camp because I wouldn't be able to breathe without my medicines.

For some American Jews, the Holocaust is our holy of holies. Auschwitz is our version of the crucifixion, and we approach it, the idea of it, with horrified awe. We imagine what would have happened to us if our grandparents or great-grandparents hadn't immigrated to America in the early part of the century. A friend of mine, a journalist who is hard-bitten (and Jewish), said to me once, Don't you wish you were alive in Europe during the war, so that you could test yourself? No, I said. Still, the Holocaust is my automatic reference point to many things—if it's really cold outside I think about morning roll calls in dark dead winter in Poland in the death camps. I can't imagine how cold that must have felt. If I'm doing squats in yoga I wonder how many I could have done if I had a gun or whip at my back and I were emaciated. These are very short, quick thoughts that I can't help. I don't verbalize them for the most part. Although I did write a book called *Holocaust Girls*, about people (like myself) who identify with the Holocaust too much.

That's why the term is a household word now.

(You mean it's not?)

Though I think about death a lot, I still can't fathom what life would be like without me in it, the way, when I was younger, that I couldn't understand how the school day could go on normally when I was home sick. *If* I die, people say, as if there's a doubt it will happen. I wonder about people who go to live in nursing homes, if life seems meaningless to them because they know it will end soon. I've always thought that people in nursing homes should be harnessed to write letters for Amnesty International. Others have pushed for combining old-age homes with day care for kids, and that makes sense. I've always felt like I'm part of the stream of Jewish history, which makes me feel less alone in the world, as if there is a place for my memory, the memory of me, to reside. Certain rabbis have been known by the titles of their books; the title became the guy's name, so that two, three hundred years later, when you mention the guy's name, you're really saying the name of his most famous book. I would like that.

When I was in a college a guy in my dorm, a hippie wanna-be, asked me if it would be enough for me to live on a commune and write just for the people in the commune. And I thought, No, though it seemed egocentric and impure to say No. You move from that question to, Would it be enough if five people read you? Then four? Then two? Then no one? Even Emily Dickinson sent her poems out for other writers and editors to read. But mostly she stayed upstairs. Kafka had his coterie and was known in the equivalent of our literary-magazine world. In his famous speech and essay "Poetry and Ambition," Donald Hall chastises poets for ambition—the ambition to be famous, to live the poet lifestyle, to churn out book after book. Instead, says Hall, you should aim to be as good as Dante. But if Dante hadn't published, how would Hall be able to name him as a standard?

Today I had a lump in my throat most of the day. That is what I call anxiety. That is what I felt throughout high school and college and after, during two dozen years of talk talk talk therapy and insight therapy and diving-down-deep-into-your feelings therapy and transactional analysis (I'm OK, you're OK—remember that?), and vitamin-nutrient therapy and aloe-vera-capsules therapy and a no-fermented foods regime, and no refined sugars and no alcohol, and acupuncture and little drops of allergens to put under the tongue with a needle-less syringe, and feminist/not-so feminist therapy, and finally the thing that got rid of the lump was Prozac. It was prescribed by the M.D. acupuncturist who'd tried Eastern and other cures on me. It worked. And its cousins in the SSRI family. To this day. Except if I don't get enough sleep, or if I drink a non-decaf latte without enough food to balance it. (Today I didn't get enough sleep and our literary magazine intern so kindly brought me a latte first thing in my morning.) Or if my body gets too used to the medley of Prozac relatives. The technical psychopharmacological term for that is Prozac Poop-out, according to my Bouncy Shrink.

 I didn't meet Linc until I'd been on Prozac six months. I tell him he's never seen me in my feral state. He's seen enough of my moodiness, so he gets the idea. He says. Once, years ago, an acquaintance (one of those people who thought law school was the answer and—surprise!—hated being a lawyer) wondered aloud why it was that so many people, especially women, need these pills to get through their lives, much less their days. She thought that the social environment was the culprit. Her view is feminist, and Marxist, both lenses that I like to use, but I don't think the patriarchy is putting the lump in my throat. I wish I could blame it for that.

 I can blame it for my non-participation in sports—that, and asthma. Linc always reminds me that it was Nixon who brought us Title IX (equality in sports) and the EPA. A Democratic Congress helped. So let's tip a hat to Tricky Dickie. One easy cause of my tension is the continual persecution of the Jews. But not all Jews are as troubled and worried and tense and anxious as I am. I have an overdeveloped flight (as in fight or flight, although I suppose there's also freeze) response, which may have been a boon, from Neanderthal time onward through pogroms. How sly Mother Nature is, though, to have given excessive flight to a person who gets asthma when she runs. Mother Nature makes Tricky Dickie look like...a third-rate burglar.

 Linc says my current anxiety is from, well, you know: my diagnosis.

February 4. Jews, Death and Taxes

For a couple weeks I'd been trying to reach an out-of-town friend who had a double mastectomy and reconstruction about five years ago. I'd sent her e-mails but hadn't heard back. She called today, and said that her workplace is clamping down on spam so maybe the breast in the subject line relegated the messages to the trash heap. She said M.D. Anderson Cancer Center in Houston, the town where we grew up, has a very good website. After we talked I Googled and found the breast-cancer page then clicked on the link for a guide for Jewish women about heredity and breast and ovarian cancer. All of a sudden on my screen was a picture of one of my mother's good friends. She'd died of ovarian cancer several years ago. Apparently her family has set up a foundation at M.D. Anderson. The sight of her just caught me. I knew she'd died, but I'd forgotten. My mother has a picture of her on her dressing table shelves, along with family pictures. I know she'd been torn her up by her friend's death. Why did the picture on the screen affect me so? I can't figure it out. I guess I'd expected to find generic information on the site, and there was someone from my personal past. The second picture was of the woman's daughter and granddaughter. I didn't recognize the daughter at first, though she used to be one of my sister's elementary-school friends and I remember the time she came on a picnic with us and got her tongue stuck on a popsicle. There was lots of information about genetic factors in breast and ovarian cancer and the higher incidence among Ashkenazi Jews (such as myself and my mother's friend and Gilda Radner and my family members who had breast cancer—three cousins and an aunt). I can say I was shocked because the cancer hit close to home, but how much closer to home can it hit than my own breast? The real answer may be that Death was hitting close to home. I was looking up my own diagnosis and there on the screen was the picture of my mother's dead friend. That doesn't seem to be all of it, but I will ponder it.

I don't know if this breast cancer has made me more weepy or if it's merely because I ran out of one ingredient in my anti-anxiety cocktail and did without a dose of it last night.

◆ ◆ ◆

Sunday we went to a small Super Bowl gathering. There was a commercial for hair dye featuring Sheryl Crow, and I thought but didn't say, She had breast cancer. Stage 1. On CNN.com last year she said, "I think faith is so important....for me to know that God had me in his hands, I never felt alone." Would she have said the same thing if she were dying of cancer? Or would she say that God had had her in his hands but had dropped her?

At the little party I talked to someone who'd had breast cancer about four years ago. It turns out she'd had a mastectomy, with reconstruction performed by the plastic surgeon I'd met with. She liked him and his work very much, and showed me her breast and scar. I said I thought her torso looked familiar from the doctor's scrapbook.

During the football game I repaired two sweaters and began reading *Bathsheba's Breast*, with its gruesome descriptions of mastectomies. The author, James S. Olson, began the book after he was treated for cancer of the hand, at M.D. Anderson; eventually his left hand and forearm were amputated. He reported that Sam Houston's wife had had breast pain and then surgery at home without anesthesia. The doctor offered her whiskey, but because she was a teetotaler and had gotten her husband to give up the bottle, she wouldn't take a drop of alcohol, even for medicinal purposes. Instead, during surgery, she bit into a silver coin. The author surmised that she probably had mastitis, a benign condition.

February 6. Austro-Hungarian Empire /Breast Grid

Linc and I left the house at about 6:40 a.m. for my MRI-biopsy appointment to check out the calcifications on my right breast. The left is the one that has to be removed. The sky was pink over the lake. I knew it was sunrise, and I knew I'd seen sunrises before, but I couldn't remember the last time. I try not to get up during the single-digit hours. I thought of the Hungarian playwright Ferenc Molnar, who was a night owl. One day he had to appear in court for a deposition. He got up in the morning, went outside and started walking to the courthouse. He was amazed at all the people on the street. He said: Do they all have depositions to make?

Molnar was born Neumann (Jewish, of course). And of course even a sunrise would make me think of Jews. You don't hear about him any more but his play *Liliom* was eventually transmogrified into Rodgers and Hammerstein's *Carousel*. During World War I he was a soldier for the Austro-Hungarian Empire and his dispatches appeared in *The New York Times*. Here's a headline, from March 11, 1915: *Shot Like Rabbits As They Climbed: Hungarian Novelist Describes Russian Attacks in the Carpathian Snow.*

◆ ◆ ◆

This morning I'd been looking forward to (well, that's going a little far: I was curious about) finding out how a surgeon goes about doing a biopsy with the help of an MRI. When I went inside the MRI last week I lay on my stomach on a mattress/gurney with a cut-out rectangle for my breasts to hang through. My head was facing left on a pillow. I couldn't imagine how a surgeon would do the biopsy: lying on the floor and looking up at my breasts, scalpel poised like Michelangelo's paintbrush? All was revealed today, though I was asleep for much of it. The staff kept talking about putting my breasts in a grid. From what I could tell, the grid was like a plastic basket that strawberries come in, with little squares formed by the criss-crossed lines. It attached to the cut-out rectangle. So I lay down on this mattressy thing, my breasts caged in this basket, and my head not on a pillow but face down against a face cradle like massage therapists provide, except it wasn't comfortable. The surgeon sat in a chair next to me, and she performed two core biopsies along the outside of my breast. They would send me back through the MRI from time to time, I think to make sure that she was digging in the right place. This is what I think she did: Put a needle in, took it out, put a marker in its place, then sent me back under to make sure the marker was in the right place. At least that's what it sounded like in my early-morning haze.

Afterward I went upstairs to the Breast Floor for a mammogram, to make sure that two markers had been embedded in the right place during the biopsy. (As I write that, I cringe at the word *embedded*. I've noticed how we use it all the time now, because of the embedded journalists with troops in the Iraq war. Is accepting the jargon the first step toward accepting the policies? Probably.)

♦ ♦ ♦

Tonight we were cleaning up the kitchen after making a stir-fry and Linc said to me, I don't want them to hurt you. And he cried. I'd hardly ever seen him cry and I wasn't sure at first that he really was. He looked a little like Walter Matthau when he cried. And then he stopped.

February 7. Telling

    The cashier at Trader Joe's who asks, How was your week? Do you say, Well, I had my first MRI, and I'm going to find out if I have cancer in my second breast?
    The good friend of a good friend you run into who asks how you are, and you say, OK, and then, Well, I was diagnosed with breast cancer. She says she'll do whatever she can, but there's really no reason for her to do anything because you haven't been in touch, and though she means well she doesn't drive. But you didn't want to lie to her and say, I'm OK, I'm fine, and let it go at that. Because, you said, your mutual friend might have told her already, though you know that he is the ultimate in discretion.
    The barista you see every day who says, What's new? How are you doing?
    The neighbor who says, How are you?
    Everyone who says, How are you? The ones who know and still ask, How are you?
    How are you? You don't know. You think you're OK. You consider this the calm before the storm. The time when you are still intact, still with your left breast intact, which will probably be gone gone gone down some swirl of medical waste. The time when you have little slits and scabs on your breasts from the core biopsies, the time when you say, My breast has a black eye, knowing from your teaching that you are employing an indirect metaphor. The time when you think about telling. You e-mail this person and that, you know that this person will tell this one, you think of ways to keep from springing it on people. What you write on the subject line of e-mails: Me. Bad News.
    You tell your yoga teacher that you won't be able to lie on your stomach tonight because of your biopsy and she says, Oh, but everything's OK, right? and you say, Not really. There was a tall blond chiropractor who was in the advanced yoga class after yours, she was known as the yoga goddess because she was so lithe, and then she had cancer and poof she died. It went to her brain. You suggested naming the yoga room after her but it became clear that rooms were named only after people who donate money.
    But this is about not telling. About not telling Amelia, your ex-best-friend, whom you used to call every morning at 10:00 to share dreams. Actual dreams. As in, Last night I dreamed that... You shared the other dreams, too. They were the same: to be famous writers. Instead both of you were bitter, obscure writers fighting for

the same things: publication, jobs. And over the years you brought out the worst in one another.

    Do you tell Amelia? But you're not dying. If you were dying, would you tell her? What would you tell her? That you are dying. Hello, is that you, I'm dying. What should we do? Will you have to be nice to me now? Which isn't fair. There was tension between the two of you: she was impatient, you were resentful, she was resentful, you wanted too much of the same things, you both had a scarcity mentality, thinking the world was not big enough to give both of you what you wanted.

    Her mother died and you heard about it from a friend, and you sent her a note. And she wrote in a magazine about losing her mother and you were jealous, really, of the published essay. Because every piece in every magazine must be written by you, and you alone, and every book written must be written by you alone, because there is not enough, never enough. And every time you think you're ready to talk to her you feel that squeeze, that never-enough-she-doesn't-deserve-anything squeeze inside you.

    You took a quiz the other day called the Belief-O-Matic. According to it, your beliefs are in line with Buddhism. Which is sort of axiomatic these days for liberal Jews. But how can you be a Buddhist when you have so much raw and deep resentment and not-enoughness in you? Where is your acceptance of life as suffering? Where is your compassion and how will you cultivate it?

February 8. I Am Milked

You can be, too. You can try it at home. Put cream on your nipple to soften it. Cover with a plastic see-through Band-Aid. Over that, lay a warmed purple velvety bag filled with stale-bordering-on-rancid flax seeds. After ten minutes have someone come in and wipe off the cream with a cloth, roughly but nicely. I'm clearing away dead skin, she'll say, like a facial. Then get her to massage the nipple, from just outside the areole, then closer in. Have her put a little suction on the nipple and apply pressure. Then watch as 4cc of thin yellowish liquid comes out of your nipple. She'll collect it in a tube.

If you do it at Fancy Hospital, you'll receive $50 in the mail in a couple of weeks. If you do it at home, no telling.

It's not really milk—this will not qualify you for a new line of work as a wet nurse.

Yes, this is what I did, as part of a study to see if there's a relationship between breast cancer risk and hormone levels in nipple fluid. When I was first asked to participate, I was hesitant, but then Linc said, It might help someone. I told this to the physician's assistant who was massaging (the proper term, not milking) my nipple and she said something like, Yeah, sometimes husbands say smart things. I said loyally, I have a very good husband. I haven't had him for even three years yet; it seems way too soon to joke about him in a general oh-those-husbands way. Especially when he's been so nicely accompanying me to Fancy Hospital.

Even more February 8. Benign!

The right breast ((o)), that is.

The left one will still have to go.
Maybe I'll have a farewell party for it.
And serve scoops of peach ice cream with cherries on top.

February 9. Doing Well

People say I'm doing well. They say I sound good. I joke. I don't think it's denial. But do people in denial admit they're in denial? On the phone a friend said something to the effect that everyone hates hospitals. But I don't. You might find it all interesting, she said. I think that's right. Which brings to mind the Chinese curse, of course.

(May you live in interesting times.)

When Jesse, son of my close friends Barry and Sharon, was diagnosed with cancer and then was in remission and then back in the hospital, I didn't mind visiting. Visiting felt like being in the middle of time standing still. Because you were doing nothing but you were supposed to be doing nothing. But visiting. And trying to give succor. To him, to his parents. And of course it was frustrating and heartbreaking because there was so much you couldn't do. A friend of mine went through a hospital volunteer chaplain course. First he followed a chaplain around and then he had his own patients to visit but he was frustrated; he didn't get to know anybody. He'd rather work in hospice. Where you are doing something. You are helping facilitate a journey. Tonight Linc and I saw *The Painted Veil* (a toss-up between that and *Puccini for Beginners*; of course we chose the movie with the dying spouse) and it did seem so comforting for Naomi Watts to be there by her husband's side. Comforting to him. And maybe to her.

I still haven't figured out mortality. We know we're here only for an eye blink of time but everything is so important to us because the eye blink is all we have. So it matters what color car and shoes and cauliflower we buy. (I saw cauliflower last week in creamy yellow and pale green, and both were cauliflower, not broccoflower.) It matters that our actions should help others of our species live well (whatever that means) and for the entire course of each person's allotted eye blink, which the ancients put at three score and ten. It matters that we read the ancients because it makes us feel connected and immortal through what I think of as *chewing* on the immortal. Here, chew on this. Learn Greek and Latin and Aramaic and you will taste the past. You will inhabit it and it will inhabit you. The oldness of the idea of the body of Christ in the wafer (not what I mean, I don't mean inside the wafer, like the stripper who waits inside the cake before jumping out), the oldness of the belief that the body *is* the wafer, and the wafer, the body—is what gives the wafer its magic.

(Says this Jew.)

Why don't we all learn to read Sumerian and hieroglyphics and the Dead Sea Scrolls, why don't we all carve out the aleph-bais on the nearest flagstone? Why do we keep looking forward, ahead, beyond? They might forget us up there in the future. There is no there yet in the future. It's all here, it's all already gone before us.

(Says this non-mother.)

In the beginning was the Word. (Say the Christians.) In the beginning was the void. (Say we.)

Then light and dark and wet and dry and hot and cold and names. Adam, meaning red, meaning earth. The notion of Adam and Eve naming the animals: What fun! What a delight! To call it a rhinoceros because it looks like one and know that everyone else forever more will call it that.

Adam and Eve opened their eyes and stepped into the future. (But if you're the Original Pair, where else can you step? Can you find a tutor to school you in the ways of the void? Step back, folks, away from that void, nothing there, folks, nothing to see. Move along, move along.)

Die defending the Torah because others died defending it and others will die defending it. And then you are calm in knowing that the memory of you, the memory of your name and possibly your being, will be preserved in the memory of those who study Torah. (I am writing this on the Sabbath, we drove a car to the movie, we did not pray.)

I meant here to explore the notion of not being so upset about the cancer. Is it because I feel I deserve to die? I have always felt I did not deserve to live, because my lungs are weak, because the tubes and passageways leading into and out of the lungs are weak. Because I am defective, have always been defective, I did not deserve to live. I have always felt that. But I think that I am not so upset because nothing has happened to me yet. The surgeon doesn't even bring a sharpened pencil to our meetings. A few people poke a few holes in me and push and pull at me but nothing has happened yet. I have not lost a breast, I have not been told that the cancer has escaped beyond the lymph node guards, or is spreading itself down my bloodstream, I have not been zapped and poisoned. I am whole.

◆ ◆ ◆

I met Barry and Sharon in 1985 at their going-away party for my friend Robin from grad school who was leaving town for a fellowship. He didn't come back and I took his place—I got his part-time teaching gig and I became friends with Barry and Sharon. Back then, they were dual-income-no-kids. Through them, I learned that you can make a literary life in the city, consisting of teaching here and there, and writing, and working for no pay on a literary magazine. When my mother met Barry on a trip here, she was relieved to find that someone who was smart and charming was living the same kind of non-traditional life I was; this precarious existence wasn't my own invention. I've lived a mile from them, then four tiny blocks, and now just down the alley. I'm a block from Wrigley Field and they're across the street from the stadium and three doors down. I like the neighborhood despite the Cubs fans and their requisite bars. The L is close, and there are little stores and restaurants and coffee houses, handsome brick courtyard buildings and two-story graystones with little gardens in front, and also hundred-year-old frame houses (like Barry and Sharon's), and people walking their dogs and I feel generally safe at night.

Once when I still lived a mile away, I had an apartment sale and felt afraid after receiving a strange phone call. I called Barry and Sharon, and Barry and the twins—Seth and Jesse, about three years old then—came over to protect me. When I was depressed in the 1980s and 1990s, I would come over (their door is always open, as in unlocked open) and sit quietly in the middle of one of the dinner gatherings they were always having and let the cheer and camaraderie wash over me. They published a short story of mine in 1986 in *Another Chicago Magazine*, and I won an award for it. Sharon brought me into her writing group around then, and we've stayed in it ever since, though she defected for a short time. We've celebrated birthdays together, sharing a surprise party once, and more than a dozen New Year's Eves. We've put up their guests and vice versa. We all apply for the same grants and awards and publications but are (mostly) happy when one or the other receives money and praise and print. Sharon has published two books of fiction and has won lots of awards. Barry is a biographer and poet with a number of books.

Jesse was diagnosed with a rare sarcoma in 1999. He died in 2001, not yet fourteen. I was a pallbearer. By then, Barry was limping a bit. Sometimes people took his stumbling for drunkenness. It was multiple sclerosis. It got worse. And worse. He used to ride a bike with his cane wedged in it somehow so that he could use it when he dismounted. Then he started using a walker that had belonged to Linc's father. Then he got a scooter. And various wheelchairs. They put in an elevator. Sharon teaches at a university about two-and-a-half hours away and is gone much of the week. We tell them what they should do about getting help for Barry, and Sharon tells us how we should rearrange our furniture. Sharon is small with thick red hair and much energy. She has three degrees in writing and one in print-making. She's lived in a yurt and crossed Afghanistan on horseback and keeps in regular touch with her waitress friends from the days when she was a college graduate who didn't know what was next. Barry is salt with some pepper with a beard at times and he drives his scooter in the street instead of the uneven sidewalk, and he rides it on the L and buses and he uses it to run over feet and into walls. Both were married once before. When we're with people who didn't know him Before, he and I like to emphasize what he used to be able to do. He wrote an essay about it: The point is, I ran. Like you. I jumped, stretched, danced, did everything a body does, and more than many.

He built a house by hand with his ex-wife. He tells everyone that his condition is a preview of coming attractions.

Both Sharon and I like to find and use clothing and furniture that's been discarded in the alley. She grows vegetables and flowers and has a compost pile and often paints the inside walls of her house. Barry is also small but he's dead weight, hard to lift and carry. He can still type and use his hands and arms some. His voice has gotten quieter and weaker and he reads and reads and is more disorganized than he was Before, which was considerably. I'm almost as messy, but I still have the use of my limbs. When Jesse was in the hospital, they brought liquor into his room and we had to be shushed by hospital staff. Sharon is older than I am and rides her bike with much more vigor. She loves to play bridge and Boggle and Scrabble and tennis. We are used to Barry being the way he is and are mad at him for becoming like this but of course we're mad and frustrated by the disease—and we know that it's only going to get worse.

February 11. Activism

Tonight our friend Bill came for dinner. He and his wife Dorreen and Linc and other friends were all college-educated activists who worked in the steel mills in order to revolutionize the working class. (Once they succeeded in that, they went on to other jobs. Joke.) Bill works for the steelworkers union and is a Costumed Activist. My term. Like a costumed hero. He organizes protests that often involve the wearing of costumes. Several years ago in order to protest the policies of Fruit of the Loom, he targeted the CEO. The CEO was on the board of the opera, so our friend got a number of people to dress as recognizable opera figures and they stood in front of the opera house, playing Wagner and leafleting as people streamed in. I would like to be a Costumed Activist. I have been one a little bit—once in the days of Ladies Against Women (feminists pretending to be non-feminists in order to show how silly the opposition was) and last year through Code Pink. What I like about Code Pink is that the organizers insert fun into the protests, which are about the serious subjects of war in Iraq and social justice. Last fall we dressed as washerwomen and gathered in front of Rep. Dennis Hastert's office to ask him to clean house and resign as Speaker. There's the same anti-Establishment sense of play or street theater that the Yippies employed. Back in 1967 Abbie Hoffman and his crew tried to exorcise evil spirits from the Pentagon and to levitate it. They organized the ill-fated Festival of Life in reaction to the Convention of Death that was the Chicago Democratic Convention in 1968. If only Daley had allowed them to sleep overnight in the park.

Could this sense of protest-fun be harnessed in breast cancer activism? What would such activism be? Getting more women to get mammograms? That's nice, easy, mainstream, doesn't target anyone as the Villain. Except if you look at disparities in the quality of health care in this country. Of course. But that's so much more difficult.

"Of all the dire health issues in the city, perhaps none is more troubling—and mystifying—than the black-white disparity in breast cancer mortality, which grew from a crack to a gap to a chasm over the course of two decades," Shane Trisch writes in *Chicago Magazine*. Experts told him that poverty and systemic racism (surprise, suprise) were the root causes of disparities in black-white health.

◆ ◆ ◆

Which brings us to joy. I agree with Barbara Ehrenreich in her essay "Welcome to Cancerland" that there's too much treacle out there about breast cancer—positive attitudes, what my cancer taught me. But there is something to be said for joy. Her latest book is on collective joy. I noticed that the Association of Writers & Writing Program's conference (which I'll have to miss because of impending though not-yet-scheduled surgery) will have a panel on creative nonfiction and joy. Enough of memoirs about trauma and sorrow and addiction.

But we do not need breast cancer to remind us of our mortality or to remember to savor each moment. That's what we have therapy, and meditation, and religion, for. And just day-to-day living.

More February 11. Public and Private

In *Bathsheba's Breast* I'm reading about William Halsted, the creator of the Halsted radical mastectomy at Johns Hopkins, and I suddenly remember that my great-grandmother's sister had cancer (breast?) and was treated at Johns Hopkins: a strange frisson of public and private. How to explain? That here's an outside reason, written in a book, for something that was a part of my family story. Each piece of information makes the other more real. How intent they must have been to get the very best treatment.

I think about this for a few days. I have my cousin (the cancer patient's daughter) on tape from 1990 talking about moving up to Baltimore to be near her mother, where she was being treated. So I was right about that. But it turns out it was throat cancer.

The four people on the tape—my cousin, her sister and brother-in-law, my father—are all dead. The most recent death was my cousin's sister, at ninety-seven, in 2005. She was vibrant and blunt, had friends of all ages, especially lots of non-Jewish friends (a rarity in my family), played the piano, knitted her own clothes, had pierced ears. The last few years when I would go home to Houston, I would call to say hello and she would invite me to come over and pick out what I wanted of hers. I have some earrings, a German plate from her in-law's family, a silver pasta server. Her earrings are heavy, so I don't wear them too often. We do use the pasta handler (one of those claw-like things), and think about her when we use it.

I don't understand the power invested in inherited things. I have my paternal grandmother's carved hardwood table (because no one else in the family needed a dining room table) and chairs and buffet, my other grandmother's stone-topped coffee table, shiny wooden desk and a red upholstered chair, and a hokey painting of a boy and bearded man, presumably a bar mitzvah boy and grandfather, who wears a beatific and benevolent smile. It may be that same old thing: we think of them when we touch or see the objects, and we feel connected to the past, and we think about how the objects will survive us, and, we hope, go to someone who remembers us.

Halsted died in 1922, so he probably never saw my great-great-aunt. He was a pioneer of surgery, introducing rubber gloves to hospital practice, formalizing the medical residency program, advancing anesthesiology. He brought fame to Johns Hopkins, and so my great-great-aunt went there for the best treatment. My father grew up in Laurel, Mississippi. When he and his siblings were sick, his mother would take them on the train to New Orleans, the nearest big city, about three hours away. When I was diagnosed, my mother said she would go anywhere with me, to M.D. Anderson or the Mayo Clinic.

I have a second opinion scheduled for tomorrow at Plain Hospital, which is supposed to be very good at breast cancer treatment, and I am waiting to get an appointment with a much-recommended second surgeon, who is Surgeon to the Stars (or at least public figures, according to his website). The only hospital the surgeon works with is Plain. He doesn't take insurance, because, I presume, he doesn't have to in order to reel in the patients. Linc is appalled that I am actually thinking of switching hospitals, not just looking to confirm Fancy Hospital's recommended procedure. If you keep futzing around, he said last night, the cancer could go to your lymph nodes. I do have invasive cancer, but it seems less than aggressive, from what the surgeon told me. She said it had been growing for about eight years. There was no urgency in her voice, like: We have to do this today. Not long ago I was so sure I wouldn't have reconstruction at all, and now I'm wanting to have a Very Good-looking Breast. Vanity, vanity.

(And I must add that I'm lucky to have fabulous health insurance from Linc, who works for a union, and that my family was lucky that it could afford to go to the best places. And that Halsted's radical mastectomy outlived its usefulness; pioneer breast cancer activist Rose Kushner campaigned to replace it with the total mastectomy, which is less extreme and less debilitating.)

February 12. Confusion Sets In

Today we went to Plain Hospital to see the Much-Recommended Surgeon there in his office with industrial carpeting and artificial plants. He said virtually the same thing the Fancy surgeon did: Need a mastectomy on the left, up to me what to do with the right. He would support me whether I wanted a prophylactic mastectomy on the right or not. I want to keep the right breast.

One thing he said that was different from Dr. Fancy was that he would remove a whole level of lymph nodes under my arm. She, on the other hand, was planning to perform a sentinel node biopsy, which is a way of isolating the node most likely to have cancer, removing it and sending it to Pathology to see if it's malignant. This preliminary check happens while you're still on the table. The node gets a more thorough analysis later, one that takes three to four days. The problem with this, the Plain doctor said, is if the node is found to be negative at first, but then, after more analysis, it's shown to be positive, the surgeon will have to go in again and take out more nodes. He'd rather take out the first level of nodes and feel around to the second level while he's in there, and can see if the second level looks suspicious. The problem with taking out those nodes is you can get swelling in your arm. I was confused and when we got home I called Wendy, who was one of the people who had recommended him. She said he and another surgeon did a sentinel node biopsy on her, but reminded me that she had stage 0 cancer and I probably have stage 2. Linc is sure that the surgeon said he doesn't do sentinel node biopsies, not just that he wouldn't recommend one for me. I consulted the Bible, aka *Dr. Susan Love's Breast Book*, and it seems that a sentinel node biopsy is the thing to do, unless a surgeon isn't skilled in it. She also warns that if the lumps are in different places, the sentinel nodes might also be in different places, and therefore one node biopsy wouldn't be adequate.

But Dr. Fancy didn't say anything about my lumps precluding a sentinel node biopsy. I will have to ask her.

I don't want to ask her. I don't want to do more research. I don't want to do any of this work. I don't want to try to understand about different kinds of receptors and look at cut-away drawings of ducts and lobules and vessels. I don't want to read about steroid antiestrogens and aromatase inhibitors and GNRH agents. I don't, but there's no choice. I also don't want to curl up and ignore all this while the cancer grows and spins through my bloodstream and lymphatic system. I told Linc tonight that I was upset and he said, Finally!

February 15. Prepare

A new study shows that men who've had vasectomies (such as Linc) are more likely to suffer from a certain kind of dementia where, say, you can still garden but you can't think of the name for tulip.

Get ready for an onslaught of late-middle-aged male mimes.

More February 15. In the Office of the Plastic Surgeon to the Stars/Following the Lump

The office of the Plastic Surgeon to the Stars was near Fancy Hospital in an old building with seemingly endless arcades in the lobby. The office upstairs was deliberately decorated, pleasingly so. Some original art in bright colors, a red and blue animal poster in the kid section, everything horizontal with clean lines. But it wasn't fancy. The ivy at the end tables was fake. While I waited, a sleek woman with very short hair was leaving her appointment and getting some face creams. She looked about thirty-five, like an Audrey Hepburn without the waif eyes, and I wondered if she had gotten a face lift. She had a lacy white knit shirt, dark pants, and a long dark coat that hung straight down to mid calf. I had come in with my puffy down coat, plastic bags on my shoes to keep the snow from leaking in, and four layers on top under the coat, and silk long johns beneath my corduroys. How did she keep warm? I assumed she hadn't taken the subway, as I had.

The doctor seemed like he'd been a nerdy science kid in high school and had grown up to become someone fluent and skilled. He measured my breasts across and in between and up and down—in centimeters, which he pronounced *sontimeters* for some reason. He did the measuring in a room for kids, and there was a sign on the wall about the patient having to pay for splints and bandages, and I realized he must do a lot of surgery after accidents. There was a brochure about prosthetics.

In his office he showed me the tissue expanders, which I hadn't seen before. Imagine a large, flat, round piece of soap. Then imagine that it comes in a soft plastic skin. Now magically remove the soap and you have a tissue expander, with a little hole in it. Magically again, and painfully, it is put under your pectoral muscle, then filled through the hole, at intervals, with salt water, to expand your tissues. When you're expanded enough, that plastic comes out and a durable insert takes its place via outpatient surgery. He had me handle the silicone-filled insert, which was soft and more natural, and the saline one (filled with aqua mouthwash), which didn't feel as if it were as thick and viscous inside. He was pushing for the silicone, but I didn't want it. He said I could decide later.

Then he showed me some before-and-after photos. I thought they looked better than the ones the other plastic surgeon had shown me. When he looked at one picture, he said, I could have done that better. He seemed so serious about his sculpting, and he talked about what he'd learned about letting the top part of the breast be flat, and ways he had of making the bottom of the new breast rounder. Through stitches inside, here and there, he said.

I decided I want him to do the reconstruction. The problem is he doesn't have privileges at Fancy Hospital, which is down the street from his office. He said it wasn't possible (I pretended I was joking when I asked but I wasn't) to wheel me from mastectomy surgery at the hospital into his private surgi-center. But he said I could get the mastectomy and come to him later, after chemo/radiation. I'd been told it's easier to get all done at once—the tissue expander put in while you're still under—but I liked that idea of waiting. He said the breast surgeon could leave on the extra skin instead of cutting it off, but that it didn't matter. How quickly I went from No-Reconstruction-Hear-Me-Roar to getting a new breast installed by the Best (as I perceive it) in the Business.

I've also been meaning to lose weight and if I did this after the reconstruction, the natural breast would become smaller, but not the artificial one. So it would be better to postpone surgery until I'm as trim as I want to be.

Two surgeries! said Linc. But I like the idea of faster recovery now. I've always been more into immediate gratification than he is. I hope I won't regret this. I also like the idea of living without the new breast for a while, just to check out what it would be like not to have reconstruction. I can always decide to just let it alone, au naturel. Which of course it isn't. And I don't want to get a tattoo over the mastectomy scars, like Deena Metzger, in the famous photo of her naked with arms outstretched. A tattoo would hurt too much. Though I'm willing to go through the procedure to get a nipple twisted from the new breast and to get that tattooed nipple-color. Under anesthesia. Local.

A friend of mine who had a double mastectomy said the hospital lost her nipple sample, so they didn't know what color to make hers. She decided on the same color as her husband's nipples but now she says that shade was too dark, and the nipples show under her clothes.

February 19. A Filling Without a Sandwich

I am a member of the Sandwich Generation—Baby Boomers (mostly women) who are caught between taking care of cranky teenagers and creaky parents. Except I have no children and my surviving parent walks the mall five days a week, lifts weights in her morning exercise class, goes to more movies and lectures than I do, and still sends me money—for my birthday, Chanukah, Valentine's Day, and whenever she makes a withdrawal from a limited partnership, in some financial transaction I don't quite understand. She doesn't need me to send her checks or to help her understand Medicare Part D. (For this I'm grateful. And I'd probably pass my mother's questions on to Linc, who explained it to his mother.) Now I am the one going into the hospital for the second time in less than a year, and she's the one flying up to take care of me.

On the phone Sunday she asked me if I needed her to do anything. I said, tentatively, If you're going shopping...are you going shopping...? Because she is a shopper. Not a clotheshorse but a lifelong shopper and comparer of merchandise. She is comfortable shopping. And as she strides through the mall she goes into the stores and sees what's on the racks. She said, Yeah, and I said, Maybe you could buy me a robe—because my two robes are terry cloth and I think they'd be too heavy to wear in the hospital bed. But she'd already beat me to it. She'd bought me a silky robe and a washable one and another one, and is bringing them with her, and I can choose any or all, she said, and she also bought me a button-down top, and my sister has approved of the purchases. I mean I just realized that most of my tops go on over my head and that I hardly have any that button or zip, and that I probably won't be able to raise my left arm for a while, and she's more prepared than I am.

What I'm trying to say is that my mother still takes care of me and by rights she shouldn't have to, and she's twenty-eight years older than I am and is healthier. Cancer-free. She is thinner and more moderate in her habits. I am faster and stronger and my hearing is better. I could beat her at mall walking, as well I should.

I feel like I'm complaining. I don't want my mother to be sick and feeble. My friend Dan is almost sixty and he says he's never grown up because he never had children. To parent (well) you must sacrifice and think of others—who are helpless—before you think of yourself. I have never taken care of anyone in that way. Linc and I have, I suppose, a mutual caretaking pact, but he's not helpless (except when he's trying to find something in the refrigerator).

Do I feel guilty bringing my mother out of retirement to take care of me? No, because she's not flying here to be my full-time nursemaid. It's only for a week or so. And she likes it. (What kids always say when they're pulling too hard on the dog's tail: But she likes it, Ma!) Really, she does. She likes feeling needed. Am I feeling guilty for having a mother capable of taking care of me? For being pleased that she wants to? Guilty because I'm not taking care of her. She doesn't need help. I researched hotels for her last night and then she called and said that when she made her plane reservation, the agent offered her a good rate (This price won't last, he told her) on a hotel. She'll pay for her flight and for her taxi and hotel. (She doesn't stay with us. She prefers a hotel.) I feel guilty—most of all, I guess, because having a healthy seventy-eight-year-old mother to help me after my mastectomy is a luxury. And luxury, by definition, is an indulgence.

February 20. Heading for Loss

I had a friend, a jokester, who used to open his wallet and ask if you wanted to see his pride and joy. Then he'd pull out a card with a picture of Pride floor wax and Joy dishwashing liquid. For many years my pride and joy has been right there on my head. Friends would say they recognized me from afar by my very thick, wavy hair. In junior high I didn't appreciate my hair. I considered it frizzy and in need of straightening chemically by Curl-Free, and then physically, by a process called wrapping. The method was passed down by older female friends and relatives, like a folk custom. You needed long bobby pins and a clean, empty orange juice can with both ends removed. After using shampoo and creme rinse (conditioner had not been invented, or rather, christened), you would towel-dry your hair, then comb out a section from the top of your head and wind it around the orange juice can, pinning it with the bobby pins. Then you would take the rest of your hair and wrap it around your head.

The theory—yes, this process had a theory—was that the larger the roller you used, the straighter your hair would be. The juice can made for a very large roller. But the largest roller of all was your own head. We needed many bobby pins for this. Then after wrapping your head tightly you would sit under your hooded hair dryer and talk on the phone for the two hours it took your hair to dry. This is why we washed our hair only once a week.

I don't talk on the phone much to my friends now. E-mail seems to have replaced both long letters and long phone calls. I used to carpool with my school friends, see them before and after school and during lunch, then at night talk to them on the phone. And then write them notes to give them the very next morning.

Somewhere in my twenties, probably when Cher's hair-do changed from curtain-straight to curly, my hair turned from high-maintenance to low. Instead of complaining about my hair, I became vain about it. I was proud, though I had no right to be, that curliness and body were things that others strove for and that I achieved effortlessly. Strangers would ask me what I ate to get such thick hair. Women grooming themselves in bathrooms would compliment me on my waves and curls. On the other hand, when a college friend of mine brought me to her parents' for Christmas dinner, her very WASPy mother looked at me carefully and said slowly, Your hair scares me.

My own mother has threatened, when I'm visiting her, to cut my hair in my sleep. My hair is what hers would look like if it were left to its own devices, which it isn't. Ever. Linc is always after me to cut it so he can see my face. So he will.

February 22. A Nervous Laugher

I have become a nervous laugher. I told someone I work with, at the place I will call Smart University, that she should meet with my student teaching intern by herself, though I would normally want a three-way meeting, but I didn't think I could schedule it because—lower my voice, move in closer, laugh a little—I'm having a mastectomy February 28.

I hate nervous laughter. It seems so fake. It seems to be covering up. It seems to be negating what you're saying. I don't want to be a nervous laugher. I remember talking to someone a few years ago about her mastectomy and she was all barky nervous laughter. It put me off. But I am doing it. I'm getting a part of my body cut off, ha-ha. If the cancer has spread I could die, ha-ha. I know that laughter is close to crying, I know that people's faces can take on similar expressions laughing and crying, I know that people say: I didn't know whether to laugh or cry, and: We laughed till we cried. Do people ever cry till they laugh? We laugh nervously. The Frenchman in the famous Liberation of Paris photo—or is it a newsreel? He looks like he's laughing but he's crying. Or vice versa. Sometimes we laugh in recognition: Hey, I do that too. But why does that make us laugh? When you do a book reading before a big crowd, the nervousness and anticipation of the crowd makes a little shudder run around the room, and everybody laughs so readily. It's easy to make a happy, willing crowd laugh. They want to laugh. They need it, to let off steam, from their waiting, their wanting. The nervousness of all being together, chairs set up in rows, side by side. All the raggedy breathing. Maybe it's the potential danger of the crowd that makes us nervous. Note the side exits. Leave bags at your seats and walk silently and calmly... A retort to the calm. We are animals that need to make noise.

The Auschwitz smile. That's what I call a certain type of survivor smile—a frozen smile that has nothing to do with and everything to do with what the survivor is relating. A smile to keep out the horribleness of it all. A smile that keeps some of the past at bay. That keeps the past from rising and twisting and striking again and again, as the voice of the survivor is telling the story once again. First we had this and then we didn't and we had no food and we had typhus and they rounded us up... The death and the dirt. The unnecessary loss. There was no reason for the loss. A madness to it all. A madness that made no sense but cut a swath of terror.

Madness, craziness. The mad are laughing crazily. At nothing. At you. At me. Voices that aren't there.

My junior year abroad I was in love with a guy named Leo and we planned to meet in Rouen, the place where Joan of Arc had been burned at the stake. His train was late. I waited and waited at the station, searching each new arriving crowd. I remember one man, frozen in my mind maybe because he looked like that Frenchman at Liberation—he was standing in the middle of the waiting room and at first it looked like he was pissing but he wasn't. A bottle of wine had broken and he was holding it before him and it was flowing out and he was crying, his face contorting as if he were crying.... Years later when I described it to someone, he said, Sounds like he was drunk. And he probably was. I remember that moment going on and on, the wine flowing and flowing, all around him, making a mess, and I was waiting forever for Leo to arrive, and when he did he said to me in our little hotel room, I feel like you expected me to come here and say I love you, and I demurred of course, saying, Oh no, not at all, but it was true. And he said, You're not fun like you were in the summer, and that was true. I felt like that French man despairing in the middle of the depot with his wine flooding out of his control. I was depressed and didn't know what I was doing in France. And I was in France because I was depressed at school and didn't know what I was doing *there*. There should be a way you could freeze yourself for a year or two when you're twenty and then you could be defrosted and jump up and know what you wanted do with your life, so grateful for the warm blood flowing in your veins.

In the car listening to the radio the other day Linc cried because the mascot from his undergraduate school is being forcibly retired. He knows that Chief Illiniwek is racist but he was a symbol of the four best years of Linc's life. He loved going to all the University of Illinois games. He loves hearing the fight song. He was part of some student fan organization that sat as a group in the stands and held up colored paper in a pattern. My college life was more like the one described in my new favorite book, *Cancer Made Me a Shallower Person*. Author and artist Miriam Engelberg depicts herself in college: *I can't wait for finals to be over next week! Then I'll be able to enjoy life again.* One week later: *Hooray! We're done. I feel great! What a relief.* Two weeks later: *What's the point of anything? We all die in the end anyway.*

There is always the void.

Let's laugh to cover it up.

Uh oh, fell into the manhole. Our laughter wasn't thick enough to cover it.

When I was in grad school I interviewed for an internship at the *Miami Herald* and thought it went well. When I'd been working at the paper for a while, one of the editors who'd interviewed me happened to say, That was a terrible job interview. We hired you despite the interview, we hired you because of your writing. And I'd thought the interview had gone well—because I'd laughed. I hadn't realized it was all nervous laughter. So I pretended to him that I'd recognized how bad the interview was. But I'd had no clue.

I was looking for Engelberg on the web today and I found out that she died—October 17, 2006.

February 24. The Party (In Retrospect)

  A few days before the Farewell to My Left Breast Party, I received a package from my friend Vera in Ann Arbor—a Hershey's Kiss larger than my head. The note with it: This is not a kiss. Oh, I figured, it's a breast. Why hadn't I ever noticed that breastal shape before?
  Vera took the train in for the party. Sharon came over early to help me prepare the food. She brought small cream puffs and added candy nipples to them. We made breasts out of tomatoes and topped them with mozzarella nipples. We sliced chicken breasts. We spread regular-sized Hershey's Kisses around the dining room table, now that we recognized what they resembled.
  I found that when you invite people to a pre-mastectomy party, they show up. Even those with small children. The kids were so young that they didn't notice that most of the food had nipples. Posey brought her daughter and son-in-law who were visiting, though he'd been hesitant, having never attended such a party before. My friend Mitch wasn't comfortable with the idea and had told Sharon he thought I wasn't taking my cancer seriously enough. But he showed up, and relaxed enough to sit down and prop up his feet.
  I talked to everyone—about what I'm not sure. Probably about my surgery. Everyone told me how well I looked. I felt giddy. I was going to go under, but not yet; I was going to be cut, but not yet; I was going to be bald, but not yet. As my friend who had bladder cancer says: The thing about cancer is you feel great until they start treating you for it.

February 25. About a Day in Which I Buy a Mastectomy Camisole & Fail to Sway an Alderman*

The nurse at Fancy Hospital had e-mailed me, asking if I wanted a mastectomy camisole. I looked it up online and it seemed like a good thing. It's supposed to be smooth against your incision, protecting it from the outside world, and it has a pouch where you can put the drain(s) that are attached to your incision. I told the nurse I would like her to write a prescription for one. She left it for me at the front desk on the Breast Floor. Friday I retrieved the prescription and also—lucky me—picked up a free (!) pink emery board from a basket at the counter.

What is the purpose of a pink emery board? To remind you to have a mammogram when you're sawing down your nails? In general the pink ribbon thing is supposed to make you Feel Feminine even though you've lost the outward manifestation(s) of what men think of as feminine in this country. Thank you, Hugh Hefner. Though we can't blame Hef. He took his obsession from his repressive childhood, and it just so happened to be the same one as the rest of mankind in the "free" world, and maybe everywhere else.

I had imagined a mastectomy camisole as a pinky-peach frilly slinky thing with adjustable slip-like straps and lace on the top. It is not. I got it at a back corner of the hospital gift store. The breast-cancer products are in back, sort of like a bookie operation hiding behind a legit business. The camisole looks like a white tank top but has elastic underneath the breastal part. Inside is a Velcro band where the drain pouch attaches. The straps aren't even adjustable. There is something so depressing about the camisole. It's called a post-surgery camisole (*Designed for comfort and function*). It looks medicinal, like the white shoes nurses and nuns used to wear. The pretty, blond square-jawed woman on the package has her head impossibly to the side toward one shoulder, though she's still facing forward. She looks defiant and come-hither. Her hair is parted on the left and pulled back and she has a scoop of hair flipping on her collarbone. I suppose this is supposed to hint at asymmetry. She is standing in a doorway with beige curtains and a white lamp behind her. She does not look like she just endured having a body part cut off under general anesthesia. The camisole comes in S, M, L, XL and XXL and you have to get it sized to your hips because you step into it. You can't put it over your head right away because you're not going to be able to move your arms up. It comes with a falsie and with batting so you can stuff the empty side.

What is it that's so depressing about this, besides the $56 I forked over for it (reimbursable by insurance)? Its genericness and ugliness. The lack of adjustable straps. Its one-size-fits-all, Iron-Curtain-country-like, Army issue-ness. It reminds me of undershirts, which I never wore, which some grade school girls had to wear instead of bras. It reminds me of the stretchy material of my first "training bra" I bought in fifth grade. We knowingly called them status symbols and bought them because everyone else was buying them. I didn't need a bra at eleven. I don't need a bra now.

The camisole is not like any camisole you would buy voluntarily. I guess it reminds me of the dailiness of the cutting and scooping and sewing that Fancy and every other hospital does day in and day out, one breast after the other, bring on the next one, hup hup. Praise the Lord and pass the ammunition. A mastectomy is a singular event in a woman's life and it's just ho-hum everyday in the life of the surgeons and nurses. As we lie on the gurney with tubes and monitors attached to us, we are not, as the rose said to the Little Prince, *unique au monde*. We are dead to the world, all blood and tissue. We're all just hamburger, says my friend Fred, who is married to Garnett and is a scientist.

And tumor. Don't forget tumor.

◆ ◆ ◆

I went to the alderman's office to buy a stack of parking permits. In my neighborhood, visitors need to stick a twenty-four-hour permit in their windshields in order to park legally, on most streets. When this first started, it cost $1 for fifteen permits, and they were undated. You could use them indefinitely (though each one only once) and you could buy two packs at a time. Pretty soon it cost $3 for fifteen, and the permits were good for a year, and now it's $5 for fifteen, and you can buy a pack only every so often. I said to the woman at the counter, I'm having surgery and expect a lot of people to come over, can I buy two packs? She said, We only sell one at a time. I said, I know, that's why I asked you. She said, You have to ask her—indicating a woman standing next to her, dealing with another constituent. She said it as if she were saying, You have to jump through a hoop of fire while juggling and turning three flips while whistling show tunes, recent Tony-winners only. I then laid my card on the table: I have cancer. She remained impassive. The other woman remained busy with someone else. My customer-service gal relented; she said I could come back next week. Implying that she would pretend she didn't recognize me and I would be allowed to buy another stack even though I was supposed to wait longer between purchases.

I have a friend who says he's tried to use the HIV-positive card before. It doesn't work that well, either.

* *So it wasn't really an alderman, but his minion.*

February 26. The Bad Girls of Cancer

Tonight was my last yoga class with two real breasts. I thought about it as we lay face down on the floor to do our leg stretches. We did a lot of back arches, too, and I wondered when I would be able to do them again. I was excited that my Bad Girls of Breast Cancer T-shirt came in the mail today so I could wear it to yoga. The front has a big black X on it over my left breast, so I thought that was especially appropriate. I ordered it from Breast Cancer Action, and I like their attitude. My politics are aligned with theirs, as far as I can tell; they criticize the mainstream Pink Ribbon people for being so corporate-sponsored, and they want to get at the environmental causes of cancer. I don't know if their method of going city by city to ban certain chemicals is the best way to go. I don't honestly know the best way to go. They're based in San Francisco, and are apparently a force there.

You don't have to go far to find criticism of the Pink Ribbon people. Our Bodies Our Blog noted Feb. 1 that Susan G. Komen for the Cure, which is named for the founder's late sister, spent $1 million for advertising. That paid for billboards with photos of T-shirts worn by women's torsos (no heads). The T-shirts say: *When we get our hands on breast cancer, we're going to punch it, strangle it, kick it, spit on it, choke it and pummel it until it's good and dead...* and *If you're going to stare at my breasts you could at least donate a dollar to save them.* I agree that this new campaign or "branding" sexualizes breast cancer. But you can't blame Komen for making breasts sexual. Linc says the ads are aimed at funders, which is true. Barbara Ehrenreich covered this ground in her essay "Welcome to Cancerland": *...breast cancer would hardly be the darling of corporate America if its complexion changed from pink to green. It is the very blandness of breast cancer, at least in mainstream perceptions, that makes it an attractive object of corporate charity and a way for companies to brand themselves friends of the middle-aged female market.* The I Blame the Patriarchy blogger is blunter: *Komen, it can't have escaped your eagle eye, is the author of those asinine, pink-visored "Race For The Cures" as well as that most pernicious arm of the megatheocorporatocracy responsible for turning breast cancer — which used to be a vile disease that kills people but is now a sweet little personal struggle that gives middle aged white women the golden opportunity to grow — into branded "awareness."*

I usually oppose the Establishment on principle, whether it's supporting pink ribbons, high heels, or war. I like being angry at the Pink Ribbon people, but wonder if my anger is misdirected. I remember how angry I was at the Cold Blonde, the inept radiation fellow who called me to say that the biopsy was "positive," never daring to utter the word "cancer." I was irate, and at the same time wondering if I was blaming the messenger. I disliked the fellow for being awkward and defensive and shifty. I dislike the corporate-studded races for the cure, and marathons for AIDS and bicycle races for MS, because I don't think they raise enough money and they are set up to make the participant Feel Good. But isn't sugar-coated philanthropy better than no philanthropy at all? Isn't it better that a percentage of the take goes toward research instead of 100 percent of nothing? But what kind of research? I don't know for certain; Breast Cancer Action publicizes research on the link between cancer and pollution and other human-made perils, like pesticides and plastics additives. BCA also studied the side effects of new drugs.

The tiny groups should be allowed to criticize the big group, the humongous group, for becoming so blindsided by its own dog-and-pony show that it loses sight of its original mission. It becomes impure. It's hard to be big and successful and pure.

Was it ever pure? I think Komen was founded in grief, and I think that was pure.

◆   ◆   ◆

In yoga, my Garnett thought my shirt said The BALD Girls of Cancer. In time, in time.

February 28. Stiff Upper Lip

Is your stomach churning? a friend asked. She'd called yesterday to see how I was doing the day before getting my breast cut off due to a disease that could kill me. My stomach wasn't churning. I wasn't in turmoil. I wasn't trembling. I was calm and fairly cheerful.

I haven't cried for a while. I've always been an easy crier and I've never thought there was anything wrong with crying. I've cried at work, on public transportation, on the street, probably in restaurants, possibly on three continents, almost-sort-of in two job interviews. But I haven't cried much lately. I remember feeling disdain for a woman sitting outside the biopsy corridor at Fancy Hospital, holding ice to her breast and crying. And I'd never felt disdainful of crying before. But I felt, I'm not going to let them see me cry. Who is *them*? Hospital staff? The world? On the other hand, I'm not consciously trying to remain calm.

I started today to feel there was something wrong with me for not feeling terrible. Do I have a death wish? Did I leap from denial to acceptance in one fell swoop? Do I see the diagnosis as a black-humored punch line delivered by Fate? I admit, I've checked out from the library the only legitimate book of Holocaust humor I know of, *Laughter in Hell*—and what's more, I thought the book was funny. Not joyously funny, but dark cackly funny. It was full of satire and irony by people who were living through a terrible time. Some making fun of the Germans, some of the situation. The essence of the Jewish joke, after all, is that a smart, weak person is in a helpless situation.

So I am a living Jewish joke. My father used to say that the hypochondriac's tombstone says, I told you I was sick. All this worrying about everything, and here I am with a malignancy. Three tumors, or else one big one that's made up of three smaller ones.

Quick, a joke, which may or may not have been in that book: Two German Jews are in Paris in the late 1930s, having fled Berlin. They're sitting at a sidewalk cafe and see a group of French soldiers march by, barely in step. Ach, says one derisively, ours are so much better.

More February 28. The Knife

I *will* be having a sentinel node biopsy. My surgeon has performed hundreds of them, if not thousands. Linc and I surmise that the doctor at Plain Hospital just plain doesn't do them.

More February 28. More Knife

Will my world finally cave in on me when I wake up tonight and see the bandage covering what used to be my left breast?

March 1. I Have Returned

I am home, we had a good dinner (a million times more nutritious than anything the hospital served), I'm not in much pain, I feel a little weak but OK, the lymph node was negative (preliminarily), of course the hospital staff woke me up every two hours, I'm wrapped in an ACE bandage and haven't seen the incision yet, I have blood draining from the incisions into two drain tubes that end in two bulbs and I can't figure how to hide them under my clothing, Linc has a cold so won't sleep with me, my student Cory and his family sent me beautiful tulips—purple, yellow, red and white.

March 2. Drain Bulbs

At the hospital, I thought it would be impossible to learn to *strip* the drains and empty the bulbs. This is what the contraptions are, as far as I can tell: Two thin plastic tubes are stuck inside the incisions and at the end of them are soft round plastic containers that remind me of perfume aspirators. They're the size and shape of a larger-than-chicken egg, only flatter. Blood flows from the wound through the tubes into the bulbs, and twice a day I'm supposed to pull out the little stopper of each bulb and pour the contents into a jar marked off by centimeters, measure the liquid, then write down the amount. You bring the log of the liquid to the doctor on Tuesday, who decides whether it's time to remove the tube-and-bulb system. Allegedly the blood will stop and then straw-colored liquid will replace it. I think that's lymphatic fluid. The stripping consists of pinching the tube near the top with the fingers of one hand and then pulling on the tube with the other, to bring the blood down through the tube and make sure any clots in the tubes are eliminated. I didn't believe the nurse when she said I would be doing this at home, but I've done it a couple of times and it's not so bad. It's odd that the blood is so—red—and bloody. This system, I suppose, is so much better than having the blood soak the bandages. The only problem is that the bulbs are bulky and show under my clothes.

Right now I'm wearing the mastectomy camisole that comes with two little inside pockets. Linc is very I-told-you-so about the camisole, which I objected to because of its name and plainness. You put the bulbs in the inside pockets. I'm wearing a nice black robe my mother brought me from home. She bought and brought me a black warm-up suit—a knit material with pants that tie with a string, and a top that's like a shirtwaist, all buttons. She also bought me a robe that zips up and has Asian people printed all over it. For a long time I didn't like wearing clothes with people on them, but I don't mind any more. I don't know why I changed my mind about this. She also bought me a lightweight light aqua robe that zips down the front. She has been very comforting except today when snow panic set in. She had never seen so much snow in her entire life, which she's spent in Texas. Snow like this in Houston would bring the city to a halt for a couple of days. It's nothing for us, here, but she kept watching it fall from her hotel room windows, and said everyone out in it was forty-five years younger than she was and bent over from the wind. She was afraid to go outside. She has osteoporosis and of course doesn't want to fall and break her hip. We got her to take a cab here at 3:00.

She called Linc when the cab arrived, and he escorted her inside. Now she is on the phone negotiating a rate for a few more days at her hotel downtown. She has a reservation for a hotel closer to here, but she's afraid it won't be warm enough, and there's no indoor coffee shop or restaurant attached.

I haven't taken a shower yet. I'm planning to do that later today, and will unwrap the ACE bandage wrapped around my chest. And I'll see the incision. I'm surprised and pleased that there's still some of the curve left on the top of my left breast. Because of the bandage I'm pretty flat on both sides, which makes it easier to get used to things. The surgeon said the incision won't be flat, there will be rolls of skin, because she saved skin for the later reconstruction. There's an enterprise I've found online that sells T-shirts that say *Under Reconstruction* on the front. Yikes. There's also a woman who paints with her breasts and donates the profits to breast cancer research. Her line of T-shirts and stationery is called Breast Buddies, and her designs consist of different pairs of colored blobs decorated to make cherries and bumblebees. I can't imagine anyone buying these except Hooters customers. I'm sure if I looked, I'd find guys who paint with their penises. It's bad enough that cats paint.

More March 2. Looking At It

I looked at the incision. To do that I rolled down the camisole and the ACE bandage. There is still some curve to my breast. How much is swelling, I don't know. There are angry stitches on the edge by my underarm and sunken-in stitches about three-fourths of the way across the breast, making the breast look smooshed in, like it's been in an accident. It hasn't been; it's been in an on-purpose. Not as horrible as I thought. I put the bandage back on and then replaced some gauze as protection, between the skin and the mastectomy camisole.

I'm going to call it my Soviet camisole; it's unlovely and utilitarian and looks like it was designed by a committee way way before perestroika.

March 3. The Angel

I just read *Cancer Vixen*, the graphic memoir, and it is in color and hardbound, and the author is alive, and it's very odd that her mother goes to chemo with her and never her husband, and she tells the oncologist she needs light chemo because she can't lose her hair because of all the super-beautiful women who are always after her husband, who owns a chic restaurant. And she loves fancy, expensive high-heeled shoes. All reasons not to like her. I admire nothing about her except her work ethic. She is a reporter-cartoonist, taking camera, tape recorder, sketch pad, and notebook with her to her cancer appointments. Her book scares me; she makes me afraid of the horribleness of chemo, the cold in your veins, the fatigue, the nausea, the fatigue, the very long needles, the pain in your hand where the nurse sticks the very long needle, the fatigue, the weight gain, the $3,500 shot you have to get if your white blood cells are languishing, and the way that shot feels like it's filling your whole body up with concrete.

I don't want to be her. I want to be like Miriam Engelberg, author of the black-and-white and crudely-drawn *Cancer Made Me a Shallower Person*, but she died. I cried for her tonight because she's the one I want to be like and she died. Linc asked tonight if I was traumatized by looking at my chest and I said no. It's true. It seems familiar for some reason. Something about the chest with its bruises and stitches seems familiar. Why? Is it because I've seen pictures of torture victims in appeals from Amnesty International and other groups? But I can't imagine that I've seen a lot of torture photos. Have I seen pictures of mastectomy scars? Maybe. The numbness in my smashed-in breast feels familiar, maybe from biopsies, especially the recent ones, where the specialists pushed and poked the breast. They were trying to save it, like bombing the village.

Linc imitates the stitches by pulling in his lips to form a straight line.

I love my right breast which is still there. And still banged up from the MRI-assisted biopsy.

I'm glad I don't need my chest for my job. I don't need my chest for my job but I would like to have it reconstructed because it would make life easier for me. My job is my writing. Even with chemo I'll have to work. Like I said, I admired Cancer Vixen's work ethic, and her mother yelling in the middle of the chemo room, as the nurse is sticking her daughter's right hand over and over: That's her drawing hand!

More March 3. The Bad Daughter

Today I stood up my mother— my loyal, loving seventy-eight-year-old mother who'd said she wished it was herself and not me who had the cancer. I was so frustrated with her for not answering her cellphone. She was AWOL, not answering at her hotel either and then she called me around 2:30 from the Art Institute and said she would leave the museum at 4:30 and take a cab to my condo. I went out by myself for the first time, to the little café down the street, Emerald City Coffee, just before 4:00 and stayed a while, and kept calling her phone from the café to see if she had left yet. Then I called my home phone and there was a message asking where I was, that she was in my lobby and it was cold and she was disappointed I wasn't there. I called her and got her and she said she was going to just go back to her hotel. I said I'd be right there. I was two blocks away. In the meantime a neighbor let her in the building and said she could wait in her apartment. When I got there Linc had arrived home and let her in. She kept saying she was going back to the hotel and I was angry and said I didn't want to leave her out there but she'd said she was leaving at 4:30 and I thought she would call me when she left. And last time she'd called from the cab to say she was around the corner. Why didn't she do it this time? All I wanted was a few minutes by myself at the fucking café. I just wanted to be alone and work, I just wanted to sit by myself in the café and write. That's all I wanted. It's my own fault for staying up reading *Cancer Vixen* but I couldn't fall asleep and took my penultimate Ambien and finally got to sleep around 1:30 or 2:00 and got up around 1:00 or so, but I was so angry too she didn't tell me where she was. And why the fuck did she say she was going to leave at 4:30 when she obviously didn't? She said she got to my house at twenty to 5:00. Well, you can't get from the Art Institute to here in ten minutes, even at 3:00 in the morning, much less a Saturday afternoon.

We all calmed down and had dinner and then she taxied back to her hotel. I sat down to write in my office and Linc kept interrupting me. I just yelled at him: Can't I just write? I want to sit and write. I feel nobody understands that about me. I don't want people around me all the time. I just want people to leave me alone. I don't want my mother coming here and saying she doesn't feel comfortable because of the mess. It's her fucking problem. Either come here or not. I would like this place to be cleaner, neater, but this is the place it is.

And I'm truly upset about this and not the black-and-blue flatness and puckeredness that is my left chest, because I'm not going to be upset about it, I'm not going to be like those superficial fucking girls who live for their cleavage, who won't take Tamoxifen because they might gain weight and the reason they say they can't gain weight is because their appearance is more important than their survival. I don't want to be like Cancer Vixen who just thinks about shoes and hair. I want to be like Miriam Engelberg but she died. I'm crying. I'm crying for her because the one I want to be like died. I'm so sad that someone who was clever and like me died.

I hate women who compete with other women, who slather you with compliments so that you won't notice they're competing because they feel you're too dumb to notice. Because they think they are so smart and are winning the competition, but part of their scheme demands that you don't know you're competing.

I am worried about picking my cuticles and infection traveling up to my lymph nodes. I'm worried about feeling nausea during the chemo and feeling tired and horrible. Even with the chemo I have to work. That's what I do.

March 5. Telling II

When I went to Emerald City on Saturday, Kati, the film-student barista said, Do you have a cold, or are you just quiet?

I leaned over the counter and said, Actually, I had cancer surgery on Wednesday.

She said, I didn't hear about it. I hope it wasn't anything major.

They took off my left breast, I said. This is my first outing.

At least they got it all, she said.

I said, I'm going to have chemo. I'm going to be droopy for a couple of months.

Then you'll need a lot of coffee, she said.

We laughed.

March 6. The Mysteries

The pathology report is full of mysteries, and in the exam room the surgeon says, Do you have any questions? I imagine that she's secretly hoping I don't, that's why she's standing up and not caring what my mother's name is, and not sitting down. (Our friend Bill the Costumed Activist has a sister who's a doctor in Vermont. Her employer has informed her that she spends too much time with her patients. Horror of horrors, she sits down with them.)

Linc alleges that the oncologist tomorrow will answer all. We'll see. It makes me angry that the report is deliberately written to obscure. Would it kill them to have a glossary attached? Or to double-space the report so that you'd have room to write notes? I have stage 2A, which I thought I had. I have lobular carcinoma in situ, which has a 20 percent chance of showing up in the other breast. I also have invasive breast cancer, which is 15 percent likely to show up in the other breast. Are these calculated together or separately, meaning do I have a 35 percent chance of getting some kind of cancer in the other breast? The largest tumor is 4 cm. My tumors dine on estrogen and progesterone. Without chemo, I have about a 70 percent chance of not getting cancer again.

I have to keep wearing the damn drain tubes, which hurt when I walk.

This cancer is starting to wear me down.

◆ ◆ ◆

I got a call telling me that my sentinel node was indeed negative, after the final tests. Which is what everyone predicted. This means that the cancers haven't escaped into my lymph system. When I report this to people, they congratulate me. As if I've done something wonderful.

March 7. Oncology (In Retrospect)

I didn't write about the meeting with the oncologist and his smart and attentive third-year fellow. I took notes, but I didn't remember anything that I wrote down, and for months afterward I would wonder about something out loud, and Linc would say: Don't you remember, the oncologist said...? And I didn't remember. What he said was that the normal chemo regimen would cut the chances of recurrence in half, but that I wouldn't receive one of the three standard chemo drugs because there was a danger of blood clots forming because of my platelet disorder, and that no one could say exactly how that omission would affect my chances. Also, the fellow explained that I didn't have a 35 percent chance of getting cancer in the other breast, but two separate chances.

Also, because of the platelet disorder, essential thrombocythemia, I couldn't get the blood booster shot between chemos, and so they would space treatments three weeks apart instead of two so that I could build up my blood on my own.

We all liked the fellow—he'd read my chart, he was friendly and light and calm. He lived in my neighborhood, he said, and (thanks to Google) I learned that he's Israeli, as my mother and I surmised, and that he goes to the same Chinese restaurant we go to on Christmas Eve.

We never saw him again.

March 8. What is a Meltdown?

It might be when you're feeling very very shatterable and don't want to answer *fine* when people ask you how you are and you're feeling shaky and so instead of going to your mother's hotel to meet her and your husband for an early dinner at 5:30, you go at 5:00 and lie down in her second bed and start crying and saying that everything is so hard and you hate these drains they won't take out, they hurt you and get in the way, and it's so terrible they have to start giving you poison for twenty weeks, even though the chemo man said most people don't have nausea or vomiting, and she is perfect in her mother role and says yes, it's hard, and lets you sleep till 6:30, when you have to get up and teach your 7:00 pm class at Smart University three blocks away. And so you teach your class, which isn't as lively and fun as at its best, but still has content and is hysteria-free. At the break your students put a basket at your place at the table with chocolates and soaps and colored pens and books, and you are able to be enthusiastic and grateful. Truly.

Afterward, as planned, you come back to your mother's hotel room to sleep (because your husband is sick and can't sleep with you because you can't afford to get his cold now) and watch the montage of TV you always watch in hotels: some *Friends*, some movie, CNN, Fox, actors vaguely familiar and young, mostly double entendres that aren't funny though the laugh track thinks everything is funny.

Then in the morning your mother has to leave for the airport and you leave her hotel and sit at the Starbucks down the street and read through the big pink binder on breast cancer treatment and follow-up, and wait until you're not too exhausted to walk the block to the subway to go home and go to sleep.

At home you sleep and watch TV and call back the chemo nurse to schedule your first round of it and you pause to weep while you're still on the phone, and she says, Are you OK? and you say you are.

Your husband says that someone at work asked how you were and he said you had a meltdown.

March 12. The Cancer Card

This afternoon I was walking from the subway to Fancy Hospital to get my heart scanned to see if it could withstand chemo. On Michigan Avenue a young woman approached me. She had on a cross, so I immediately assumed she was an evangelist. But her first question was, Do you live here? Usually I pass up street hawkers but I was curious. Yes, I told her. Then she said, Can I talk to you about your hair? I said, I'm going to have chemo and lose all my hair. Oh, she said, falling back.

I felt so guilty I called Linc immediately on my cell to confess. He said that no one has a right to accost me on the street, that whatever she got in return was fair. Later tonight he said, People don't have an inalienable right to sell things.

March 13. Happy

I was standing in line at the Bourgeois Pig Café. It's one of my favorite coffee houses, a place with wood everywhere and antiques for sale, and I was thinking, I want a blueberry scone. I asked myself: Would that make you happy? (The answer was supposed to be No, I don't need all that butter.) And I thought, I am happy. I feel good. I was sort of excited and scared that I'd made an appointment for later in the week to get my hair cut, by a specialist in curly hair. I'd decided I should get at least some taken off so that I could gradually get used to having no hair. So I was in the café and felt a sense of contentment. It was hot, and crowded, but there was no jostling. It was the city's fourth day of early spring, and I'd seen daffodil buds outside Fancy Hospital an hour before. I was anticipating the coldness of my iced latte.

Fancy Hospital is near Smart U, and I'd gone there after my appointments to print out some student papers. I checked my e-mail messages, and found one from a friend who'd just heard about my cancer. She said, It must be scary and terrible. But it didn't feel that way. I'd finally gotten both drains removed (they were stuck inside my body about three inches deep and poof, took milliseconds to remove) and I felt happy in my hot pink long-sleeved T-shirt with Linc's blue work shirt over it, with my Cancer Sucks button over the left pocket.

I knew at least one reason I was happy was that I had all my medication. I'd been out of Cymbalta for a couple of days last week, and it showed. From age sixteen on I was in therapy (because I wanted to be) and the therapist and I—or the group, the therapist, and I—would try to analyze my emotions and change them. Or analyze my thoughts and change them. Or dig deep into my feelings and the family dynamic to find IT, the Reason for my anxiety and worry and lump in my throat.

In the gift basket my students gave me last week was a book of linked stories by Margaret Atwood. In one of them the narrator talks about her sensitive weepy, unhappy, suicidal sister, and how finally everything changed—when she took a pill. Snap! That was it.

It is like that. I think of all the years I spent analyzing anxiety—which the pills later dissolved. Years. Years. I was at the point of not returning calls because I was crying all the time. I lost a friend for about a decade because of that. And then, Prozac. I found him again, in Wisconsin. And after Prozac, I stayed in therapy another ten years. We are so influenced by Freud, who in turn was influenced by his society, of course. The question my best professor used to ask about every phenomenon was, What question is this the answer to? What question was Freud the answer to? I think Freud was the answer to the question, How can Enlightenment principles be applied to solving emotional problems? For Freud, it was easy: The patient suffered X because she repressed an unconscious desire to do Y. You get them to talk long enough, and they'll figure that out. Narratives that illustrated the trajectory of these desires had already been mapped out by the ancients. Interestingly, Freud turned to the Greeks and not the Hebrews; he didn't give us the Solomon or Ruth complex. Though he did write *Moses and Monotheism*. He believed that Moses was murdered, a theory that was going around.

Your parents wanted a boy, a therapist with a New York accent and beard concluded when I was in my twenties. That's why I was anxious. But my parents wanted girls. They wouldn't have known how to deal with boys. Freud would ferret out the offending belief or repressed urge, bring it into the light, and poof! he would ease the person into *ordinary unhappiness*. If that person was a female, he would urge her to accept the role of the conventional bourgeois woman. Second Wave feminists criticized psychoanalysis for this, as well as for the idea that the vaginal orgasm was the only real, mature kind. Many years ago I read a well-known and sort of silly biography-as-novel of Freud and Breuer's Anna O. I couldn't figure out why the author had herself photographed on the book jacket wearing what appeared to be thick mascara or false eyelashes, and (if I remember correctly) pearls. Then I got it: She was showing us that although she had succeeded in the male world by producing a creative and intellectual object, she had managed to keep a tight hold on her femininity.

I was thinking about all this as I sat upstairs, next to an open window, at the Bourgeois Pig; I had finished grading the papers and eating my blueberry buttermilk scone. The room has red walls, a bookcase with old books, a pink velvet sofa and a fireplace with a carved mantel. Last summer in that very room I'd gotten involved in a conversation about Freud, and in so doing met a rabbinical student who (it turned out later) had gone to school with a student of mine. Three years ago, Linc and I were married here, in our fifteen-minute ceremony. When people see the wedding photos, they think we were in the rabbi's study.

Tonight Linc met up with me at the Pig at about 6:30. He was self-castigatory because he'd lost his cellphone on the L. I called his phone and a very nice guy answered, and then we jumped up to go meet him and retrieve it.

More March 13. Hair

I went to the Cancer Floor at Fancy Hospital, where blood was taken for some reason related to the upcoming chemo. I met Lora the Chemo Nurse and asked her if I would lose my hair, even though it's so thick. She said yes. I said, Is there no way it would still be there? and she said no. She told me that it was going to be gone from Day 16 after the first chemo treatment until three weeks after the last treatment. So that means from early April through late August or early September. For some reason I thought it would be for just a couple of months. The other day I got a prescription for a cranial prosthesis. That means a wig.

My hair reaches about to my collarbone. I can't imagine my hair gone or even thin. I can't imagine it but I'm also planning ahead for its predicted fall. I figured I'd send my hair to Locks of Love, which provides hairpieces to needy children. Then I wondered if a kid would want my salt-and-pepper hair. (Here, kid, the good news is we got you a free wig. The bad news is you'll be a ten-year-old with gray hair.) As it turns out, the website says: *Hair that is short, gray, or unsuitable for children will be separated from the ponytails and sold at fair market value to offset the cost of manufacturing.*

I imagine an outdoor market of hair vendors.

So my hair would qualify for donation, just so it's at least ten inches long and in a ponytail. So then that means that the first stage of my hair-shortening will require at least ten inches off my scalp. At its longest, my hair is about fourteen inches long. I was thinking it might be fun to get a different hair cut every week. I would love to have a mohawk for a week or so, as long as I didn't have to represent Smart U in any public programs. I wouldn't mind, but I think Smart U might.

Such are the travails of the non-tenured.

March 15. Heart

Today Linc and I were waiting at Fancy Hospital (this time, for his doctor) and I was looking at our palms, wondering what our life lines showed. I should get my palm read and see if the fortune teller can see the breast cancer first, I said. To test her. He said, She can just look at you. You're missing a breast.

We were waiting for a cardiologist, for Linc's hypertrophic cardiomyopathy—a thickening of the heart wall. He also has a murmur. First we had to undergo the sacrifice of Those Who Go To Teaching Hospitals: the ritual humoring of the med student or new doctor. Our fellow was slightly nervous and slim with beautiful dark eyes and lashes. He asked all the questions whose answers were probably right there in the file: age, activity (basketball 3-4 times a week, bicycling in reasonable weather), medicines, symptoms. Linc really has no symptoms. His main complaints are his two very cautious doctors—his internist, and the cardiologist his internist sent him to. He's had an angiogram (squeaky clean) and cardio tests that left round pink irritations on his chest for three weeks. His blood pressure doesn't go up much when he exercises; it could be because he's in such great shape, or it could be part of his malfunctioning heart. The cardiologist has been muttering for a couple of years about a heart-valve replacement. What Linc has is what makes student athletes drop dead on the playing field.

The fellow listened to Linc's heart and breathing. Then the doctor put him through all the same paces. (That's my main complaint about these young doctors. They basically use the patients for role playing. I told Linc I should have told the apprentice that I was feeling sore around my heart, could he take a look. Would he be in for a surprise!) The cardiologist said that it seemed Linc was OK, that to be totally safe maybe he shouldn't engage in competitive basketball; even Michael Jordan hung up his sneakers. Hard exercise carries a risk, he said, but it was unknown what exactly the risk is. Basketball is Linc's great love, his Zen, his flow experience. Linc explained that he plays with old guys, that the game isn't as competitive as it could be. In fact, they call themselves the Geezers. The doctor said that heart-valve surgery is usually performed in order to make people feel better and that Linc seems to feel good. Linc said: Somebody would have to speak more forcefully than you are now to make me stop playing basketball.

The cardiologist said he would check with the cautious cardiologist about the results of other tests, and would probably put

Linc in a 24-hour halter to follow all his heart-blood comings and goings.

On the way to the elevator Linc said, Dropping dead doesn't scare me at all. What he meant was he wouldn't mind dying on the basketball court; he'd rather be dead than languish. Linc's father had many heart attacks and that is why Linc started exercising seriously in his thirties. I am proud of him. He's more or less the same size as the day we met. I have gained thirty pounds since, and those pounds have turned me from a pear-shape to an apple, which makes one more at risk for...ahem...cancer. It seems an hour of exercise a day is one of the best preventatives. Cancer Bitch will work on motivating herself. Her heart, according to the scan she had the other day in preparation for chemo, currently has nothing wrong with it.

March 16. The Neighbor Boy

The Neighbor Boy came by the other day. This is accurate but also misleading. He did not amble by, tapping on the kitchen window next to pies cooling on the sill, and say, Howdy, Missus Cancer Bitch, I'm home for spring break and thought I'd give you a look-see.

No, this Neighbor Boy came over because his father sent him to pick up a fax. His parents, Barry and Sharon, give out my fax machine number as their own. They have a fax machine that's like blood type O-negative, the universal donor. They can send only. They could receive but each spouse has been waiting for the other to buy fax paper. For years.

The Neighbor Boy, aka Seth, rang the downstairs bell and I buzzed him up. He knocked on the door and I answered it, resplendent in my glasses and long and full Lanz nightgown. It was late Saturday morning and he said: You're taking it easy.

I have breast cancer, I told him.

He was floored. Literally: he sat down on the stairs. No one told me, he said.

There used to be two Neighbor Boys, twins that I couldn't tell apart, but then Jesse got cancer. When they were about ten I used to drive them to soccer practice and they'd sit in the back like aspects of the same person, riffing off one another. They both were gifted in mimicry and memorization and sometimes the sound from the back seat sounded like spliced tapes—first part of a speech, then word plays, things that made a sort of logic by association. One of them had mused to me once, All things considered, all kings considered, that... At the time, I couldn't tell which one it was. One of them told me more than once that I had a pointy nose like a witch's. Or maybe each said it once. I told him/them it wasn't a nice thing to say. My suspicions are it was this Neighbor Boy, the one who survived.

I learned about giving people what they want the first time Jesse was in the hospital. I asked his mother what I could do, assuming she would ask me to buy groceries, which I enjoy doing. I like wandering around the supermarket. Instead she asked me to go home and make sure that Seth wrote a paper that was due the next day. I didn't want to do that, but I did. He was smart. He is smart. They were both really smart, early readers, eager readers, having so much to say their tongues couldn't keep up with their thoughts. The paper was about pollution, and he did a good job with it. My job was to keep him on task, which wasn't so pleasant. I learned that what you want to give isn't necessarily what the other person wants to be given.

Seth is now a sophomore in college and told me about his upper-level anthropology course on drug culture. He was planning to write about the image of the drug dealer in movies of the past forty years. He was going to start with *Easy Rider* and go up through *Trainspotting*. It is tricky with the Neighbor Boy. He is temperamental and won't answer questions directly. Like a lot of kids. I think of him as a night-blooming plant. You never know when the flower will come so you have to be ready for it. I let him talk. I made comments. He told me he'd loan me some DVDs. He said, Now we'll have to visit you in the hospital.

I said, I'm already out. They didn't keep me long.

I told him sort of vaguely, I think, that I knew cancer was scary for him but that it seemed like mine was caught early and that I would be OK, that a lot of people survive breast cancer.

His twin died of cancer and his father has MS. His life has been full of loss, if that's not oxymoronic. Jesse was in the hospital on Halloween when they were twelve and I went trick-or-treating with Seth. He was on the cusp of being too old. We went to Alta Vista Terrace, a nearby block of historic row houses. We both liked it. I got to feel like I had a child. He got to feel like he had a parent with him. Once months later I was in the car with the boys and Barry and Jesse was talking about a camp he was going to for kids with cancer. Seth said, I wish I had cancer. Jesse said, No you don't.

March 17. First Hair Cut of the Year

Cancer Bitch went for her $60 hair cut Friday with trepidations and a ruler so that she could send ten inches of hair to Locks of Love, though it's a controversial outfit. (In 2002, it supposedly gave out fewer than two hundred wigs and collected hundreds of thousands of dollars.) She came back with a more sophisticated haircut and nothing for Locks of Love. The haircut will get her used to seeing her own face. Hairdressers always say this: Now you can see your face.

It was a one-person salon less than a mile straight south of me, on a street with restaurants and houses and a liquor store. The owner has long African-American-Korean hair made up of little curly waves. It was tied back. She was very friendly and when I told her about my plan to cut my hair progressively shorter, she told me about her mother's cervical cancer. Amazingly, she'd been treated well and successfully at the county hospital.

The stylist did not approve of what she called my "umbrella cut," which I've had for many years. I never saw anything wrong with having hair that got progressively wider on its way to my shoulders. Her strategy was to make a diamond cut, which means that the hair would be wider on the sides than the bottom.

She measured the strands before she cut them and said to forget the ruler, she'd just give me a good cut. The pieces on the floor were about four inches long. So I won't be donating my hair. Maybe it's just an excuse, but I'm not sure how effective any of the wig programs are anyway. Wigs for Kids' finances weren't audited by a CPA. I can't find an evaluation for Beautiful Lengths.

I think my hair looks good. It's curly all over. At its longest, it's a few inches below my ears.

Chemo starts Monday, March 26.

March 19. Covering

Yesterday and today I spent too much time on the web looking at chemo-head headgear. I don't like most turbans and scarves out there and I would want to try them on anyway before buying them. I did send off for temporary tattoos for the scalp from an outfit I found called ChemoChicks.com. The medium is henna and the design is a swirling leaf pattern. I also ordered eyebrow stencils. A girl has to plan. Sharon has agreed to apply the henna. She has an MFA in art so she should be able to integrate a peace sign into the leaves.

March 20. Gender: Hiding the Evidence

When I went for the scan to see if my heart was up to snuff for chemo, I wore the mastectomy camisole under a red flannel button-down shirt of Linc's. I didn't wear earrings because I thought I'd have to take them off in the scanner. I looked in the mirror and thought I looked androgynous.

This is the abiding mystery: Why do we need to know someone's gender? I remember in the days of the hippies, how Middle Americans would say, in accusation: I can't tell if that's a boy or a girl! The question is, Why do you need to know? Once in high school a girl looked at my fingers and exclaimed: You have men's hands! because I had hair growing on them. Hair that I must have bleached at least once when I was bleaching the hair on my arms. We bleached and shaved, a way of lying about our bodies, Adrienne Rich was writing and thinking at the time, though in my teens I'd never heard of her. It was female to shave our legs and underarms, but still shaving was something we did so we wouldn't look manly.

I've been mistaken for a male a few times. The first was in Paris where I went my junior year of college in my attempt to escape my boyfriend. Going to Europe seemed easier than breaking up. In France a person did have to know what gender another person was, out of politesse. You had to say, *Mademoiselle*, may I see your ticket? Or, *Merci, monsieur.* Or *Oui, madame.* The first time was when I was coming back to Paris from London on the ferry, in those pre-Chunnel days. I'd rolled my hair so it would be springy on the way there to visit Leo, who was spending his junior year abroad in England because he wanted the adventure, not because he was running away from anything, or anyone. I was tormented because I didn't have a good reason for being in France. Or Europe, or anywhere. He was unhappy that weekend because I wasn't fun. On the way back, my curls went flat and the ticket-taker on the ferry called me monsieur. When I arrived back in Paris it was Sunday night and I was so upset that I called—what else?—the American Embassy emergency number.

Cancer Bitch has never been afraid to ask for help. Once in college I called a crisis hotline while on a date to hear Muddy Waters. My problem, I told the counselor I'd reached on the pay phone during intermission, was I wasn't getting into the music. In Paris, unbelievably, the embassy worker on duty invited me to her apartment. (I think I'm remembering this right.) She was very sympathetic. I was very hysterical. I must have gone home that night to the French widow I was boarding with, and soon I was in therapy with a Greek woman at an American cultural center. Later that year I was in therapy with a polyglot Jewish woman originally from Romania who had been living in Israel. I'm not sure what she was doing in Paris, but France in the mid-seventies must have been more appealing than Israel at that time, with its wobbly infrastructure and rampant inflation. We mostly spoke in French. At the Alliance Française, where I was taking classes, I met a handsome Tunisian who'd been speaking French most of his life, thanks to colonialism. He became my boyfriend. I remember how surprised I was that he didn't know the word *angoisse*, anguish, a word I used often.

A couple of years ago Linc and I were on our way back from Springfield and stopped at a vegetarian café in Normal, Illinois—the only vegetarian café in Normal. I asked another customer where the restroom was and he said, The men's room is there. It confounded me more than bothered me. Maybe the guy was stoned. I mean, I was a married woman. So I had to be female!

Am I afraid that when I'm bald—whether I have a swirly tattoo or not—I'll look male? I don't think so. I'll be wearing a pair of earrings to clue in the general public. I've noticed that scarves and hats and turbans for chemo-heads bill themselves as feminine. The flowers and pastels remind me of unfashionable Easter hats. The bright prints and stripes seem doggedly determined to convince the buyer and the world that there's a female underneath the fabric. A smiling woman, if you look at the pictures in the catalogues. But the world is going to look at you and figure out that you're undergoing chemo, because no one else wears those turbans, no matter what the ad copy says. The caps and scarves are supposed to cover up our loss, hide the evidence of our treatment. Give us privacy, perhaps. The bald head publicly declares: I had cancer and I'm not pretending that I'm not getting chemo. In other words, Death has brushed me.

March 25. Why I Hate Elizabeth Edwards

Because she might die.

Because she didn't find her lump in 2004 until it was the size of a half dollar.

Because she smiles. She smiles and she is dying, the cancer is in her bones, it is eating in her bones, and though there are drugs that may stop it, that might stop it, the drugs might not work.

I hate Elizabeth Edwards because her husband John is not quitting his presidential campaign in order to take care of her, she doesn't want him to quit, she is in the race for him, for both of them. The campaign is a mom-and-pop affair, according to her. She is not working as a lawyer. She wants to work to help her husband win the presidency. She wanted many things. She wanted children in her fifties and got them. She got a husband who became a senator. Did she want that? I don't know.

She can have what's called *quality of life*. She can have a good life, she can take a pill, and another pill, and a treatment, and she could be in the 5 percent. Or 10 percent. She could live more than ten years. She wants a legacy of helping her husband into the White House, not of keeping him from it.

I do not like her husband. I heard him speak the first time he ran and he was vague and said he understood the poor and the workers because his parents had been poor and workers. He wanted us to vote for him because of that. Because of who he had been. Of what he had been born with. Nothing.

Now everyone says he is seasoned, he knows he was wrong about the war on Iraq. He is for universal health care. See, his wife is so sick and he wants everyone to have the health care that she has. This is his bully pulpit. She says, he says, they want to perform service, that's the reason for the campaign. He is not blindly ambitious, he wants to help, and he can help the best by becoming the most powerful person in the world. On earth.

They do not talk about the possible causes of breast cancer. About pesticides and pollution and that the company that brought us Tamoxifen, AstraZeneca, was part of Imperial Chemical, which produces carcinogens that have been linked to cancer. AstraZeneca sponsors Breast Cancer Awareness Month and supervises and must approve all its brochures and public relations because who knows what might come out otherwise. Elizabeth Edwards does not use words like the ones Rachel Carson might, for example, who warned us in the 60s about the environment failing us and moreover us failing the environment, and she was scorned and is now a secular saint.

    I hate Elizabeth Edwards because she didn't get a mammogram for the four years before she felt the lump. Her cancer came back after chemo and radiation, and I just had my second chemo treatment. The chemo is supposed to kill any errant cancer cells swimming around in my bloodstream. The odds are good. Elizabeth Edwards says: We are all going to die, I just know what it is that will kill me.

    Elizabeth Edwards had stage 3 cancer, a lump and malignant lymph nodes. My nodes are clear. They are shiny and perfect, doing their job.

    I am a better person because I am only stage 2A, because mine was caught earlier. I am on track. I am prompt. Though she found hers on her own, and I found mine through a mammogram. We should have joined forces; I would have urged her to get annual mammograms and she would have persuaded me to do a breast self-exam each month. We could have been bosom buddies.

    She is going to die and she is not raging. I am not raging. Because my cancer hasn't come back. Because it hasn't had time to come back. It was just removed one month ago. I am not raging, people notice that. I am not angry. I feel I deserve this. Because? Because I am fundamentally flawed. The breast cancer attached its crabby legs around me, it caught me living an imperfect life. It caught me drinking milk with bovine growth hormones. It caught me eating cheese. It caught me drinking tap water in the farm belt. It caught me because it catches one out of every seven or eight of us women. Because that is the luck of the draw. Because that is the price we pay for modernity. For post-modernity. For the mosquito fogging trucks. Fogging, that was the term. For not being the perfect athlete, the perfect vegan, the perfect organic-eater. For not being even a good athlete or good exerciser or proper vegan.

    I know that hate is fear. I hate this cancer, this strange overgrowth inside me that is against my own interests. The cancer is in her rib and her hip, breast cancer has migrated there. You can't hate cancer, it's just cells that took the wrong message, answered the wrong phone, opened the wrong letter. Cells that did not know you could return to sender.

    I have to hate something out there. I hate Elizabeth Edwards because she is not screaming, screaming: This is unfair. I didn't want this. I don't deserve this. We don't deserve this.

March 26. Chemo Begins...

...with the installation of a port attached to a tube inserted in the jugular vein. That way, the nurses will go straight to the port, instead of hunting for a vein each time I get a chemo infusion or blood draw. I hope it's the right choice. Linc has a friend at work who had trouble with her port. I wanted one because Cancer Vixen's drawing hand started getting numb from the chemo needles. And when I was in the hospital for surgery I had an IV in my hand and it hurt for weeks after.

The port-installing doctor said it would be like dental work, where you don't feel pain but you feel pressure. I felt nothing. Or don't remember feeling anything. It was quite Proustian—awake and dreaming at the same time. The nurse said I also talked about flying in dreams.

Then we were off to the Cancer Floor for the chemo. I thought it would be a room with three to five lounge chairs and women in varying stages of side effects. And then one day we would find out melodramatically why one person never came back. Instead, I was in a private room with a regular examining table and a rocking chair, and the nurse gave me Ativan and some anti-nausea potion through the IV and then she pushed in the medicine, as she said, the Adriamycin in a syringe attached to the tube attached to the needle in the port. I couldn't feel much. I could see the Adriamycin, which is red. Then more saline. Then it was over, after maybe thirty minutes.

We left with three prescriptions for pills to fight nausea. Linc and I picked them up later at the drug store. Two medicines are mandatory. One is optional. I asked the pharmacist if he knew anyone who went on chemo and didn't get nausea, and he just looked at me helplessly.

But I am hoping. I had some Indonesian ginger chews sent by a friend in Oakland and I am wearing the anti-motion-sickness wristband my sister sent me.

My sister also sent herself, from Houston. I haven't spent much time with my sister alone, not for years and years. She is cheerful, easily amused, calm and not irritable. She's a learning-disabilities diagnostician in a school and we talked about special ed and autistic kids. She's taking a class and she had to finish a paper for it, and fly home tomorrow to hand it in. We also talked about her plans to hold both Passover seders at her house, for the first time ever. When my father was alive, he and I led the seders, using parts of a feminist Haggadah. After he died in 1991, I went back to

Houston every year and led at one or both seders, adding new material, constantly checking out new Haggadahs. I always thought the seders there couldn't go on without me. I think my constituents likened me to Castro: It seemed I would always be there, and I would never name a successor. This year I'm not going home; seems like too much coming on the heels of chemo.

Meanwhile I keep asking myself if I'm nauseated. Like poking at a bruise and seeing if it really hurts. Right now, I'm OK. Let's hope.

March 29. The Stores

I've been wandering around the neighborhood, scouting out stores that look like they might sell hats or wigs. Last night I went to Hollywood Mirror on Belmont, which had mannequins in the display window wearing red, black and white scarves. As if they were just waiting for Cancer Bitch, ready to tell her that scarf-wearing was fashionable. Inside, the music was blaring. There were little displays of hats, mostly berets. I don't need scarves. I don't like them. There were a few punk wigs that looked promising. I went to another store that specialized in accessories for bachelorette parties. The closest useful thing I found was a plastic halter that had three breasts on it. I thought I could wear it for my follow-up exam with the surgeon. I would put it on under the gown and say, Doctor, I've been feeling funny... Or better yet, try it on the fellow first.

It took a while to figure out what to say I'm looking for: fun wigs. They're colored, unrealistic, maybe $10. But I couldn't find any I liked.

March 31. Listening

I haven't had any nausea, but now I have this headache. It's like a sinus+tension headache and nothing helps it except, if I'm trying to sleep, Ambien. I'm afraid I'll become addicted to Ambien. I've taken it about five nights straight. I didn't know this morning if I should get up and walk three miles or sit around in my robe and read. Do you listen to your body at this time when it's reeling from the chemo? Do you rest, or do you push on because you've promised yourself to walk every day, and walking will make you feel better? Which part of yourself do you listen to? Which is the legitimate part? Which is the whiny, weepy, wimpy part that needs a push? The thing is you don't know. No one can tell me if even after the twenty weeks of chemo, I'll be cancer-free forever. That is true. And it seems stupid to be hopeful because you could be wrong. But it seems self-defeating not to be. Isn't it better to hope and believe that I'm already cancer-free, that the chemo is just to make sure, that all this will be a bump in the road when I look back on a long, healthy life? The opposite is to be the sadder but wiser girl, the I-told-you-so girl. But what is the value of being able to say I told you so on your death bed?

April 1. Two Miles

I walked two miles to the Bourgeois Pig Café. I didn't feel better or worse when I got there. I got a small decaf latte and read *A Contract With God*, the graphic novel my student Tim had sent me along with the sappiest card he could find bearing the message: *Hang in there.* The novel is so dark! Will Eisner wrote and illustrated it based on the death of his daughter from leukemia. Later tonight I gave it to Barry and Sharon to read. Sharon wanted to say something sad about Jesse and chemo and I said, No, don't say it, and Barry said, No, don't say it, and Linc said, No, don't say it. And she didn't.

When I talk about my port and she talks about Jesse's port, all seems doomed. Cancer means Jesse and Jesse means death from cancer. I saw him after he died. He was lying in his bed upstairs. He'd been dead a few hours. They didn't know what to do. He'd been alive the night before, talking to his doctor and a patient advocate from the hospital, who'd come to visit. A few of us sat around the table, the same table where we had chicken soup tonight. They hadn't known what to do. I mean, Sharon had just been trying to find clinical trials Jesse could be part of, and investigating a healer in Brazil. They called the synagogue and the hospital, which sent an ambulance, I think. Another friend carried Jesse downstairs. When Seth came home from school, early, there were his parents' friends sitting there looking at him. I think I hugged him. He said something like, It's OK. Meaning, the death of his brother was OK. Because what else could he say? He had to shrug. Because the table was filled with adults. And then two years later a friend of the family died, another young man, and the adults were sitting around the table and one of them went up to Seth and said, I'm sorry that you've lost your friend.

There is so much loss. And on the other hand, Sharon's mother had breast cancer twenty or so years ago and is alive in South Florida or Cleveland, depending on the season. Alive and with husband.

More April 1. *El Repliegue*

Today I felt better as soon as I woke up, though I'd only slept about nine hours, and the night before I must have slept thirteen. And I can't define or delineate what is better. I still had and have the jittery, run-down-feeling headache. But it didn't bother me as much. How difficult it would be for a doctor to treat me. I'd say, I feel the same, except it was bad yesterday but not today, and I can't tell you how it's different. With this sort of headache, I feel the pain as dispersed pieces of glitter floating in my head, as suspended in gel. I could say amber, but it is more like gel, soft. And I feel I can't unfurrow my brow.

I was thinking yesterday about motivation and encouragement and I thought of the *repliegue* in Nicaragua. The *repliegue* is the annual re-enactment of the Sandinistas' strategic withdrawal or tactical retreat from Managua to Masaya in June 1979. Afterwards the revolutionaries came back to Managua in triumph. I was in Managua in 1989 because I wanted to figure out how the revolution was doing, and whose fault it was suffering economically. Were its weaknesses due to the Sandinista leadership, or to US support of the Contras, who were fighting the government?

Of course, I never figured it out. I spent the summer teaching English to government health workers at the equivalent of the NIH, except it looked like a run-down elementary school and there were chickens in the yard. I was sick (*turista*) almost the whole time, and came back, my friend Sharon said, almost too thin. In Managua in late June I was so sick and weak that I decided not to go on the nineteen-kilometer *repliegue*. It was a Friday afternoon. Then I suddenly decided to join; I was lonely. I started walking and caught up with the march. I would talk to whomever I happened to be walking with. Somehow I found one of the few people I knew in the entire country, a Californian who had come to Nicaragua with the same volunteer program that I had. I joined him and his Nicaraguan host and after we reached Masaya we slept on the sidewalk overnight. In the morning we took the bus home and my friend was pickpocketed. Well, we were there as volunteers, right? To give what was needed? So what was the problem? It was in Nicaragua that I also learned how to give graciously. I had some drawing paper that a friend said his friend would like to have. He said that instead of just leaving it for him, I should write a note. And I did. I also bought someone an entirely superfluous wedding present. I should have given her American money. I still cringe thinking about it. I can't bring myself to recount the details.

What is the lesson for me, for my capitalista-individuista psyche about my experience on the *repliegue*? I didn't expect myself to join the march. No one expected me to. But because no one expected me to, I did. And I was fine. What does this say about motivation and walking when you're weak from chemo? That if people tell me not to, it's easier to motivate myself? That I'm tougher than I think? I know that often if little is expected of me, I do very well.

I know I keep hearing in my head the hearty voice of Lora the Chemo Nurse on the phone: I'm sure you'll do great. She said that on two occasions and then I asked her: Why do you think that? And she had a reason that I don't remember. Probably having to do with the improved anti-nausea drugs. And I haven't been very nauseated. Of course it is still the first week. She said I might have heartburn and I have. She said I might have constipation and I haven't. It strengthens me to hear that cheerful, confident voice in my head.

We want to predict the future. We want to be reassured that we'll be safe and happy. People who pray build an image of how they want things to be. They exhort or implore the deity to bless and take care of this and this and this. Imagining is powerful and can change physiology. So I've heard. Yet a part of me fights against doing this. It's too too...invisible.

April 2. The Fifth Question

The Four Questions are ritually asked on Passover, beginning with, Why is this night different from all other nights?

The fifth question is how and why we celebrate the holiday if we do not believe in the historicity of it, that we were slaves in Egypt, and if we do not believe in a deity; if we do not put any credence in the central covenant we read about on Passover, the covenant with God—that He told Abraham, I will make your people slaves but after four hundred years I will liberate them and they will be a great nation; that as the result of the torture of the tribe, they will emerge a cohesive group and they will have a land of their own. This is the same lesson that some people draw from the Holocaust: The Jews were tortured and burned in Europe but then emerged, liberated with a land of their own.

It has been said that modern Jewish practice is ancestor worship. We put on this ritual and set this table and bake this kugel because *Bubbe* did it. We take a little bit of the *tam*, the taste, of the holiday and swish it in our mouths a bit, and wait for the memories to blossom, Proust-like. Proust was Jewish but I don't know where his Jewishness lay. Or half-Jewishness. *The New York Times* years ago had an article about Passover macaroons; it quoted a Jewish baker saying the canned ones set off Proustian associations.

I always wanted a seder where people argued and discussed, and we did both tonight at Barry and Sharon's. But we did not get to the answer to the central questions: What does this mean? Why are we here? What do we do about the readings that we don't like? The Exodus story is true, claims the chancellor of the Jewish Theological Seminary, even if it didn't happen, just as great literature is true. The Exodus is one of our central myths. Our daily prayers (which we don't recite) mention being taken out of Egypt. I have read more than a dozen Haggadahs that try to make the story and the holiday relevant. If you do not believe, you have to think your way around so much. You have to change the *donnée* of every Haggadah and say, There is a story that our people have told, and it is not historic. Yet it has great meaning for our people and it has mythic structure. You have to qualify everything.

And after you've done that, you say to yourself, This is a holiday in my bones and blood, its cadences are driven into me. And that's why I'm here. And while I'm here on a purely emotional level, that is the reason for my return: I want to get some intellectual and moral sustenance. But all that is so much work. But to not do that is to be reduced to the level of a child absorbing a fairy tale without question, because it's so familiar.

April 3. Passover—First Day

The first day of Passover comes after the first night.

Part of the reason we celebrate/observe (Lenny Bruce said Jews *observe*, that *celebrate* is a goyish word) Passover or any other holiday, aside from nostalgia, is the longing for the belief of our ancestors. They were sitting around a seder table, just like we are, and they actually believed. At least we think so. We would like to think so?

Can we think so without being condescending?

The Hebrew word for Egypt is *Mitzrayim* (from the Hebrew *metzar* meaning *a narrow, tight place of being*). The interpreters ask, What is the narrow place that you are trying to escape from?

April 4. The Forgetting of Elvin Hayes

I have long had an image in my mind of the seder of my dreams. It's like a class of my dreams. Everyone is smart and engaged and wants the reading and discussion to go on and on. And the singing.

Our family has never had seders like that. They aren't big singers. My youngest aunt was a good singer but she died. My other aunt's second husband was a good singer but when my aunt died he went elsewhere for seder. My father was an off-key but enthusiastic singer, but he died. His rendition of *Khad Gadya*, one of the songs at the end, sounded like a football cheer in Hebrew with Yiddish pronunciation. I have not heard the like of it since. This generation of children is quiet and not show-offy. You need people with bluster to carry songs all the way through. They say that cantors are frustrated opera singers. We need frustrated Broadway musical actors at our seders.

The seders I lead in Houston are big, maybe twenty-five people, and the people are usually sitting at five different tables. That makes it hard for discussion. For a while we would go around and say who we missed, but then it got too sad. At the end of the service, we read aloud, Next year in Jerusalem. Meaning, next year perfection. In that spirit, we've written wishes on index cards and then read wishes written and saved from the year before. That got too sad, too. Then we'd talk about Passover memories, but they were mostly generic. I wrote a series of I-remembers, linked to different eras, such as: *I remember how hot the soles of my feet would get when we were walking in the desert.... I remember blisters all over my hands from the bricks for the Egyptians...* I would pass these out to everyone, and each person would read a different one aloud. Was this meaningful to my constituents? I don't know. Was it just an exercise in literary ego? The idea came from a book by Joe Brainard called *I Remember*—a standard in many creative-writing teachers' toolkits.

Sometimes we used the old books, a pre-war Reconstructionist Haggadah that featured illustrations of androgynous men wearing loose shifts. What was nice about those Haggadahs was the leader (my father, and before him, his father) would make notes, so you would see, next to the *Mah Nishtanah* (always recited by the youngest child), the name of my aunt who was now very much an adult.

I went to a seder last night in Highland Park, graciously invited by an adult student who'd figured I wouldn't be traveling to

Texas. Linc opted not to go; he was traumatized by his bar mitzvah and avoids ritual as much as possible.

Our seder leader was like a good teacher. We read through the service and he would offer tidbits now and then, such as: Every time there's a pivotal point in the Bible, there's a woman. He gave background about a famous paragraph in the Haggadah in which five rabbis are mentioned. (This paragraph usually falls, by chance, to a young reader who stumbles over all their names.) We are told that the rabbis stayed up all night discussing Passover. This is an object lesson for the rest of us, who've been through the story dozens of times: Even the greats found something to discuss. They were splitting hairs, such as debating whether *all the days of your life* included the nights, both actual and metaphorical. Another interpretation of their all-nighter is that they were staying up to plan the Bar Kochba rebellion (132-135 CE) against the Romans, who were oppressing the Jews. What our leader did last night was tell a little about each of these rabbis we'd been naming every year. Rabbi Tarfon, for example, was famous for saying, It is not your job to finish the task, nor are you free to avoid it altogether. Rabbi Joshua of Galilee was a blacksmith who was the last holdout in the rabbinical debate about making chicken *pareve* (neutral), meaning that observant Jews would be able to eat it with dairy. His argument was that chicken wasn't meat, because the biblical commandment is to not cook a goat in its mother's milk, and a chicken's mother doesn't have milk.

If his faction had held sway, the entire course of Jewish cuisine would have been completely different.

Each family has its own ways of doing things and I missed our ritual of reciting a counting song, "Who Knows One?" in English. Everyone tries to read the last paragraph in one breath. This family sang it in Hebrew, and kept going faster and faster with each added number. I also missed substituting Elvin Hayes for *El b'nai* in the chorus to *Adir Hu*. This year I realized that you could also substitute Karl Rove for *beka'arov* in the chorus. I will have to tell my people next year.

I'm thinking that discussion might not be necessary. Last night there was some back-and-forth but I wasn't champing at the bit to make one point or the other. Have I longed for robust (the current buzz word) discussion from my people as proof that they were listening? Maybe they were listening quietly all these years. It can be enough to learn something interesting. *Dayenu*.

More April 4. An Aside: Education in Nicaragua, 1989

Inflation made the value of the currency change at least every week. Every week a bus token cost more. I have still one piece of Nicaraguan paper money with three zeroes added on, printed officially by the national bank. The electric grid was unstable. It wasn't unusual for the lights to go out in the middle of class. Our room didn't have any windows. There would be certain days when we didn't have running water. Water service was rotated by neighborhood. The night before the water was going to be cut off, we would fill up barrels with water. The plumbing wasn't so great to begin with. You weren't supposed to flush anything, even toilet paper. There was a wastebasket next to each toilet for you to drop your used paper. And you'd need to provide your own toilet paper. This was in the capital city. It had buses that worked, though they were always filled beyond capacity and it was usual for young boys to hang from the outside of the bus. There were pay phones, or at least places where there had been pay phones, but every part of the apparatus had been stripped. I could never figure out where I was or how to get anywhere. The street names were informal or nonexistent and any signage was handwritten; a street or area would be named after a local resident who had died fighting for the revolution. Regular street names and numbers had been destroyed in the 1972 earthquake. My address was something like: three blocks north of the Esso station, a block from where the baobab tree used to be. There were taxis, but for some reason the drivers wouldn't turn around to pick you up. You had to be going in the same direction as the cab.

I was teaching English to government health workers, lab technicians with the equivalent of a master's degree and nearly starvation wages. There weren't photocopy machines. I'd brought copies of English exercises with me and ran the class by feel. Everyone was at a different level. The previous teacher, I'd been told, had drilled them on verbs. I'd been told in a way that made me feel I should do the same. So I did, some of the time, or I would help the students translate English instructions that came with a machine or instrument, or ask them what they had trouble understanding. They asked me how to pronounce *grocery* and weren't satisfied because they expected a three-syllable British pronunciation. I taught the most advanced student the term *I have a time conflict*, then wondered if that was idiomatic enough. He grew very attached to that sentence.

One day I went to the bathroom at work, and started to toss my used paper in the trash. In the wastebasket I saw something that looked familiar; it was an exercise from a few days before. I said to myself, At least I know that that handout was useful.

April 5. The Neighborhood Acupuncturist

In March I went to an acupuncturist affiliated with Fancy Hospital, and she seemed inattentive. Yesterday I tried out a new acupuncturist, recommended by a friend (who had prostate cancer) who sees this acupuncturist's mother in Chinatown.

The place is about a ten-minute walk from home, in a half-basement office below a brick apartment building. The waiting room is small and white with a bench with three square cushions on it, a few plants and big vase in the corner. XueHua greeted me by name from behind the counter. He looks about thirty, with wire-rims and frequent smiles. It was windy and snowing very very slightly yesterday. He wore a blue shirt with vest. I had to wait about twenty minutes.

He asked me questions and looked at my tongue. He asked how I was sleeping. (Hadn't gotten enough the night before.) I told him I had a sore throat and the beginning of a cold. He took my pulse and blood pressure. I lay on my back on the massage bed and he stuck me in my head and legs, telling me what he was doing as he did it. I'd had acupuncture before, and wasn't scared of the needles and could barely feel them. He brought a heat lamp to warm my feet. Then he cupped me. I had seen this done once before, in Nicaragua. This is how he did it: I lay on my stomach and he lifted my shirt. He took a small glass cup that looked like it could hold a votive candle, then picked up scissors holding a gauzy pad, dipped the pad in alcohol, then (behind my back) lighted the gauze, put it in the cup for a moment, then put the cup on me. It felt like a suction cup. Uh, I guess it was. The smoke, he said, got rid of the oxygen. He had several cups and put them down my back. He left them on for a few minutes. They felt tight, and hurt a little. When he took them off he said the circles on the right side were red, which meant I had more tension on that side. Cupping increases circulation and releases energy and toxins, he said..

He told me that he can help with chemo side effects. He didn't want to give me herbs because he said I already take a lot of medicine and he wants to use foods to heal.

Cooling foods cause nausea, he said, and hot ones cause headaches.

I'll meet with the acupuncturist next week to tell him how it went. Today I woke up and I was more stuffed up and my throat hurt more. I'm thinking, Well, he stirred everything up and that's why I'm worse. How we rationalize! I decided to call my regular doctor for an appointment. Got one for tomorrow. Onward. Of course when I showed Linc the red circles on my back last night he was horrified. I look like a pepperoni pizza.

April 9. The Government Knows Much

Last month I received a fat business-sized envelope from the state of Illinois. For a second I thought that it was from the Illinois Arts Council, containing a complaint about my writing the year I had an arts council fellowship.

I know, I'm both self-centered and paranoid.

It was from the Department of Public Health, and included a gift bag! (Congratulations, you have cancer. Here's a free gift!) It's an eight-and-a-half-inch square beige bag with a big pink ribbon printed in the center. On the top it says, *SHOW YOU CARE.* Underneath the ribbon it says, *BE AWARE.* All I can say is How and How? And what do you put in such a small bag?

Forgot to mention that the handles are pink.

There was a letter enclosed from the state director of public health that described a study on breast cancer. The group is trying to get a handle on why African-American and Latina women have a lower incidence of breast cancer but are more likely to die of it. (I can tell you—minorities generally earn less, and thus have poor access to health insurance and good medical care. There's a local study that shows that in 2003 the mortality rate for black women was 68 percent higher than for white women, even though black women are less likely to get breast cancer.) This new study will look at the patient's social environment, delay in seeking treatment, and type of treatment.

Today a young woman came to my house and interviewed me. I was disappointed that all the questions were fill-in-the-blank, multiple choice, or true/false. What about my unique story? Oh, I guess that's what my own writing is for. The questions centered on my diagnosis, medical treatment, confidence in my doctors, my emotional support, the safety and resources of my neighborhood, my civic involvement. It took about an hour and a half and I got $100 in cash.

Today I received a postcard from the district police office. It said that on March 30, my car was observed *...with personal property clearly visible. In an effort to reduce theft...we are asking that in the future, please secure personal property out of sight...* That must have been the night I left my cellphone on the front seat. I think this message is odd, and sweet.

Needless to say it mentioned nothing about my breast cancer.

April 10. Hair is a Woman's Crowning Glory

I am still with hair. Lora the Chemo Nurse said I would begin to shed on Day 16. Today is Day 15. I've heard your scalp starts tingling before the hair falls out.

Is it tingling? Is it? I'm apprehensive about losing my hair, afraid I'll look terrible but still so curious. Excited, even. Amazed that this thing could happen that has never happened to me before. (I suppose you could say the same thing about death. I don't think I'd feel the same way about death, though.)

I took a bath today and lost a lot of pubic hair. It collected in the hair trap in the drain. It looked like a swarm of ants.

April 11. I Left My Hair at Second City

I went to Second City tonight with a friend from L.A. and her beau. Throughout the performance I was combing my hair with my fingers and coming out with strands. I formed them into a ball about the size of a jacks ball. We were sitting in the last rows so I don't think I was very distracting. Maybe I was. I'm sorry if I was. I laughed out loud once, during an otherwise dumb sketch about four Slovenians comprising that nation's army, which was helping the US in Iraq. Then a fifth fighter came on stage, and they all yelled, Surge! The American asked what his name was. Serge! he said.

April 12. When It Falls, It Falls

My hair kept on falling out and falling out. You could see the part widen in the middle so that my scalp was visible. It is a nice scalp, pink and not scabrous, I'm happy to report. I'm sure I left a puddle of hair at my table at Emerald City Coffee. So tonight it seemed like it was time.

After dinner Linc and a visiting dignitary, Roberta of Boston, shaved my head, leaving a road of hair down the middle. I was very cranky and scared throughout. I thought it would be a quick buzz cut, but instead it was a scissors cut followed by a tedious, scraping regular razor-and-shaving-cream process, with additional judicious snips with nail scissors. We told Roberta that if she ever gets tired of being a tenured academic she should try hairdressing. She has a keen eye and is attentive to details. Good work ethic, also. She will list the haircut in her CV under Service, as an interdisciplinary project in conjunction with the graduate program in creative writing at Smart U. It will be called *Using Geertz's thick description (and shaving cream) in the acquisition of a new skill set in experiential adult education in a non-traditional setting.*

Instead of spikes I have a roll of big curls in the middle of my scalp. Still I look like a goth. I feel that I should be mean and sulky because I have a mohawk. I will have to smoke cigarettes and apply for a cashier job at Whole Foods. Will the punk kids there recognize me as one of their own and teach me their secrets? My *voisins de palier* Anand and Maureen came over for scotch. Mo said I look very young.

In a day or two the mohawk also will fall off and I will be another bald woman with cancer. Or being treated for cancer, even though the cancer has been cut out.

When my head is hairless Sharon will apply a design of leaves to my head with henna. In the middle I want her to write, US out of Iraq. Then I will just be another bald-headed woman for peace.

April 17. Men with Guns

Monday on the subway going to meet Linc at chemo, I was rereading Peter Gay's memoir, *My German Question: Growing Up in Nazi Berlin*, in preparation for hearing his lecture Tuesday at Smart U. A more accurate subtitle: Growing Up Jewish But Not Really Jewish in Berlin, and it Not Really Mattering Until the Nazis Made it Matter. Train stops, I shut the book, walk to the exit. A man standing there, looks at me and I'm thinking he's looking at my hat because clearly I'm bald underneath. He says, *Auf Wiedersehen*. I look at him and smile. Apparently he saw that the book was about Germany. It *is* about Germany, in a general and very particular way. Was he showing off his German? Was he German? He didn't look German. He was pudgy, maybe in his early thirties, with dark cropped hair. (Peter Gay's father didn't look Jewish; his non-Jewish business partner in Berlin didn't look German.) Gay's title is obviously a play on the term The Jewish Question, which was asked all over Europe in the 19th century: Could the Jew be a European? The man on the L did not ask the Jewish Question. He did not ask any questions. He assumed. I assume he had no idea who Peter Gay is. (The family name had been Froelich, meaning happy, so they changed it to Gay.) I feel there are so many layers and layers of thought and history and life and assumption between what the guy on the subway said and whatever response I could have given.

◆ ◆ ◆

At chemo, Lora asked if we'd heard about the shootings at Virginia Tech. I'd heard vaguely, Linc hadn't yet. Several years ago some young Israeli soldiers came to a local university to talk about why they refused to serve in the Occupied Territories. They were talking about how strange it was to be the US. One said something like this: If this were a university in Israel, you'd have metal detectors and soldiers at the gates and in all the buildings. And the audience laughed. I couldn't figure out back then why they laughed, and I still don't know. Because such measures seemed ludicrous? The young soldiers were bemused. Why are you laughing? they asked no one in particular, and no one answered.

Some day there will be armed guards everywhere and we will shake our heads and think about the time when we had free access to so many places. I remember when stores didn't have security guards. Hell, I remember going to Foley's and Neiman Marcus and Battlestein's in downtown Houston and just telling the clerk my parents' name and address, and being able to charge clothes.

◆ ◆ ◆

    Saturday we went to a memorial service. Afterward, an eighty-year-old cousin of the bereaved family started talking to us and looked at my hair and said, You're an artist, aren't you? You're making a statement. I didn't feel like saying, NO, I HAVE CANCER, so I said, Yeah, I'm a writer.

April 19. Head Covering

I became un-mohawked last night. I'd suspected that the mohawk was staying put mostly because of hair gel. I combed it and the mohawk came out in hunks, leaving a very thin veil of hair behind. When Linc came home from basketball, I made him trim and electric-shave the middle of my head. There were strange ridges left around the mohawk border, and I made him shave more, even though he was dead tired. Then I was mad at him because he hadn't been eager and adept, but mostly because I was so unhappy to lose my hair. The mohawk was fun, he said, and bald isn't fun.

Today I am feeling droopy because I am un-mohawked even though I am still grateful and pleased to have received two hats (one handmade) in the mail from friends. The sun is shining, the daffodils might actually recover from being cold-nipped the other day, but I had trouble sleeping last night and I want to go crawl somewhere and watch a movie. But I want to walk three miles and grade some papers. I went to the bank today to finish up some work on my IRA I'd started Tuesday and the guy there had to copy down my driver's license number. He looked at the picture and asked me (wearing a hat) how I went from the driver's license hair to a mohawk. I said, Chemo. And told him I'd lost the mohawk yesterday. Oh, he said, that's not too exciting. He seemed disappointed. I suppose he wanted to hear about a dramatic mid-life shift. Maybe he imagined getting free tickets to hear me play in a punk band. And thus his life would be changed.

April 20. Cancer is Boring

It is life-threatening but boring. And mysterious but boring. Mysterious because I don't even know if I still have it. Was it all cut out? Is this long, hair-losing journey into Chemolandia unnecessary? No one will ever know. For a mystery to be pungent we have to have a certain level of information. There is not enough information now. I can get my blood count and such, but not my cancer count. No one knows if little cells are causing havoc. Which sounds exciting. No one knows if the little cells are landing in a fertile patch and reproducing wildly. Which also sounds exciting. But is projection. The cancer cells do not have feelings. Or brains. We don't think. Maybe they do and they're thinking that humans are big brainless machines or worlds.

I am bored. I am bored of this flatland, end-of-semester, is-that-all-there-is? feeling. Let's call it the Second Round of Chemo Dropoff. Cancer ain't new anymore. Threatens to become routine and dull. Or maybe I'm just sobered oh so sobered by losing my hair and wanting to be pretty and not look like Telly Savalas but not wanting to get a wig either because... because that would be fake? expected? because it would be hot and uncomfortable? because I want to not do the standard thing because then I would be like everybody else, and as the girl said in the long-running musical, *The Fantasticks*: I am special. Please God, please–don't let me be normal.

Cancer is ordinary and extraordinary. A cell gets a little genetic or environmental jolt and off it goes on its own like a windup toy that doesn't stop or may not stop. Or may rattle and shake and ruin the whole toy shop in its crazed journey.

Boring people get cancer. Exciting people get cancer. Clods and dolts and geniuses. I'm sure people who study cancer think it's fascinating—at first. But they probably get bored too. Because they are nose-to-nose with it. Every day. Trying this and that, being very careful to calibrate and measure. Using the scientific method. Taking detailed notes. They study cancer's properties. They are trying to parse it. Adding this and this to the soup to see what happens. Or doesn't.

April 23. Notes on the Visible/Invisible

The shaving of the head, in order to make women visible, to shame them.
The continuum from voluntary to involuntary hairlessness. Look for *chemo caps* or *chemo hats* on Google and you find rosters of turbans and cloches and caps and sun hats and scarves and wigs soon you will find the Yiddish word *tichel,* for handkerchief. The Orthodox Jews and the residents of Chemolandia, both part of a market share. The Chemolandians just passing through, the pious there for the long haul. Where are the scarves for Muslim women? They don't turn up. To find them you have to look for *hijab*. And then the world opens up for you, of luxury *hijab* pins and *jilbab*s and bonnet caps, and you learn that Ikea has commissioned a hijab to be part of its sales-clerk uniform.
The shaving of the head to create instant conformity: the military, of course. The shaving of the head for hygienic purposes, to rid the community of lice. The shaving of the head as humiliation, to make the Jews/any prisoners/ just one of many. Oneofmany. In her memoir *Seed of Sarah,* Judith Magyar Isaacson describes her first day at Auschwitz. The showers. The real ones, with water. Then she is shorn and shaved and disinfected, and stands in line for clothes. Then she is rushed at a by a male inmate in a ragged blanket. It is her mother. Without hair, everyone has become male. Everyone is the same.
The medicine took away my hair. I focus on the hair, the hair, that is what is lost. We focus on the hair, the hair the hair. It begins to fall away, which I cannot help. I am help-less. So then I cut and shave it. I leave behind a mohawk, I shape the hair that is left, therefore having agency, as the PhDs would say. Then the mohawk, my mohawk, falls away. And I shave off the rest of the very thinned hairs. I henna the bare head. Thus I have agency again. I am seizing the means of —-decoration. In a way, I have chosen all, I am in control. I have chosen to comply with the medical establishment. I have chosen to take its poison. I have chosen the poison so that I will not die. I will take the draught that kills, but not all the way dead. Just a little. It just kills a little. I am a little bit dead.
My hair is dead, it falls away. Inside me, rapidly-multiplying cells are attacked rapidly. Inside there is a battle of strong versus weak. The cancer cells want to gallop away and the chemo runs after them, to stop them in their tracks. The chemo pursues. Adriamycin is red and can destroy tissue, you must be careful when administering it. If you are a cancer cell, beware beware.

It is all invisible, this raging war. The patient is told to conjure up this cell eating that cell. Strong happy cells munching on cancer cells. A Pac-Man game inside the body. Your mind will keep the score going up and up. Your mind and will.

April 24. Freedom and Development

We went out to dinner Saturday (it seems we are always going to dinner; we are; we're yuppies, I've said to Linc; no, he said, we're not Y; oh, then I said, we're nyuppies—NOT-young urban professionals) with Jack and Val, old friends of his from their organize-the-working-class years in the steel mills, and Tom, who works as a lawyer and writes books. Val and Jack were talking about Amartya Sen's *Development as Freedom,* and then Tom and Jack were talking in a sprightly, involved fashion; they were having an Exchange of Ideas. Among the five of us there were three households, and all subscribed to the *New York Review of Books.* Jack both reads it and remembers what he reads. What I am drawn to in the *Review* is the easy, familiar stuff—biographies and Holocaust and Alison Lurie on children's lit. I also like the foreign policy critiques that reinforce my own attitudes. I was happy and all to be with intellectual friends talking about a Nobel prize-winning economist, about whose work I must have skipped myriad articles, but what I really wanted to talk about was my scalp. Why, did people think, did I still have stubble? Logically, if all my hair was falling out, the stubble should be falling out, too. One explanation is that longer hair puts more weight on the hair root and thus leads to more rapid hair-falling. But still, when I ran my hand across my head, no hair came out, and wouldn't that friction against it equal the pull of long strands? We had talked about the vagaries of my hair and scalp a little bit before dinner, but I thought the subject could stand a more thorough and nuanced analysis, preceded by a summary of the earlier conversation. But no one at dinner saw fit to re-discuss my hairs, and conversation turned to other matters. Such as this story from Tom:

Army recruiters are apparently scouting the parking lots of supermarkets and the like, aiming to capture young people leaving their minimum-wage jobs for the day. Tom's nephew works at a suburban Jewel supermarket, and a recruiter approached him in the parking lot and started his pitch. The nephew listened and gave him his phone number. The nephew has no intention of joining up. He's a senior in high school bound for college in the fall. The Jewel isn't the end of the line for him; he works there because his family has a strong work ethic. This is what surprised me: He didn't feign interest in order to be mean or to be a prankster. It was instead part of a thought-out effort to protect the recruiter. The kid was afraid that the man would be sent to Iraq if he didn't provide enough names of live prospects and he wanted to delay the recruiter's deployment. He wanted to keep him safe.

He also had Caller ID so he could avoid the man's phone calls.

We ate at Caliente up the street. By chance, Lora the Chemo Nurse was at the next table. She didn't talk about my hair either.

April 24. Henna, Head and Ankle (In Retrospect)

How long does it take to henna a head? It depends on whether you read the directions first. I didn't. I went to Sharon's Sunday evening and we figured out how to use the stencil from Chemochicks.com. The process is too tedious to describe, but involved eucalyptus oil and cutting and taping paper with designs on it, mixing up the henna potion, pushing the potion from a plastic cone into a plastic applicator bottle. If I'd read the directions beforehand, I would have known that the henna paste had to sit for a couple of hours after mixing. Sharon followed the stencil and made some designs of her own, and wrote US OUT OF IRAQ on the back of my head. The henna felt cool and pleasant on my scalp. She said it was like decorating a cake, except the applicator bottle is hard plastic and required Herculean squeezing. The henna wasn't dry by the time I went to bed, so I had to wrap toilet paper around my head before I went to sleep.

The designs are quite beautiful and swirly and I feel dressed, not bald. The henna is hard and black but will flake off and be less pronounced. I am so glad I have a decorated scalp. I was in Trader Joe's tonight in the soup-olives-peanut butter aisle and a little girl said something to her father about funny hair. I said: I don't have any hair. I have designs on my head. You have to choose one or the other, I said, hair or designs. I didn't feel bad at all. I think I would have felt much more self-conscious if my head were bare.

I remember reading about a pregnant woman who sold space on her belly in exchange for Super Bowl tickets. Three people so far have suggested I sell advertising space on my head. My friend Jodi in Madison wonders if short people will be able to read the back of my head, and if I'll need a T-shirt to explain my head.

April 25. A Cancer Bitch Behaving Badly

Yesterday I went out lightly dressed and didn't mean to be gone all day, but I was. And it got colder and colder (52 degrees). Around 8:00 pm or so I walked the half mile from Letizia's Natural Bakery on Division near Damen, where I had a latte and a chocolate chip biscotto* and did some editing work, over to Ashland to get the bus.

The bus came. I got off at Addison and waited in the drizzle for the Addison bus. When I exited at Clark it was still raining. There was a Cubs game and I was going to cut through the parking lot but some young guys in Cubs-type uniforms were standing bunched up near the entrance and said, You can't go through the parking lot. I said why? One of them said, Because the players come through here and you can't get close to them. I didn't ask him why the players would be leaving in the middle of the game. He said I could take another path that was almost the same. I was so angry and cold and damp and didn't want to take an extra step. I yelled, It's raining and I HAVE CANCER!

And I turned and took the other path. It really was almost the same as cutting through the lot. I was so angry even though I was laughing at myself. I could understand how people get out of control and become abusive in public. I wanted him to recognize how stupid it was that there were five guys standing there guarding a lot from me. Me me me. I am harmless. I am a Wrigleyville resident, not some stupid fan. I live around here and put up with the Cubs traffic every year and the fans peeing and shouting in the alley and stealing our potted plants from the porch. I am wet and cold. I am one-breasted and bald, on my bare head I have written US Out of Iraq, I'm missing most of my eyebrows, I am almost home and I AM CANCER BITCH.

*Nota bene: *Biscotti* is plural only, despite what you hear and read. It means twice cooked. Thus terra cotta means cooked earth. Panna cotta means cooked cream. Or you can just ask for the mandel bread.

April 27. Cancer Bitch Behaves Badly Again

I went to Caribou Coffee. There were bags of coffee for sale with pink ribbons on them. Part of the price goes to Susan G. Komen for the Cure, which goes for—what? More pink ribbons? I think Komen should sign on with Christo to wrap every woman with pink ribbons. Then it won't matter if they have breast cancer or not, because you won't be able to see it. As long as you can't see it, it's not a problem. And when they die, the survivors can turn the ribbons into a shroud.

Oh, where was I? Yes, Caribou does sell coffee with pink ribbons with some portion going to the Komen foundation. I asked what the percentage was and the barista told me that the company had pledged $100,000 and she asked if I wanted to buy a bag of coffee, and I said no, that as someone with breast cancer I support an organization that researches the cause. Which is true but makes no sense. You think someone with breast cancer would be focused on *cure*. But I guess I'm just a selfless Cancer Bitch. I regret that I spoke to her in a tight and aggrieved tone. I think she felt sorry for me because she offered me a Caribou lottery-type scratcher card and when I wasn't a winner she kept taking out more and more cards and scratching them even though there were people in line behind me. Finally after a half-dozen cards she gave up.

May 3. The Holter (Not Halter)

We are falling apart. And Linc's employer is paying for it. Linc is taking a Holter monitor test. Not wearing a halter, as I had thought. Holter is the guy who invented the monitor, attached to Linc's belt during the day and put in a shirt pocket at night, to record everything his heart is doing and not doing over 24 hours. The cardiologists want to rule out arrhythmia, which is not good for thrice-a-week basketball players, or anybody else for that matter. Linc is irritated because electrode wires are stuck to his chest and the adhesive is itchy.

Now he is pressing tape against my scalp then pulling it off to see if loosely-held stubble will come out. This interests and amuses both of us. We are like monkeys checking one another for lice.

May 14. Prayer

Saturday Val and Jack dropped by. Jack works against pollution on an international scale and had just returned from Dakar, Senegal, with a scarf for me. It is large and red and black, anarchist colors, he pointed out, and he was apologetic that it was too large for my head. But I had taken informal head-wrapping lessons in an African import store in Hyde Park last month, and I knew how to twist and tuck. So I spent most of Saturday evening wearing a large turban. The Tanzanian kanga cloth I bought in Hyde Park has bright blue, yellow and black markings and a proverb in Swahili that says God is good or wise or something like that. I also bought a soft blue hat in the store. I still had my mohawk then. I told the store owner that I was going to lose all my hair. She asked why and I said I had breast cancer and was going through chemo. Oh chemo is not good, she said. Chemo is poison. When she realized I was determined to continue my treatments, she asked me for my name so she could pray for me.

A number of people are praying for me. As the archetypal Jewish mother says, It couldn't hoit. (This is the context in which I've heard that line: The son proudly treats his immigrant mother to a Broadway show. In the last act, the hero crumples to his death. The mother stands up and yells, Give him chicken soup! The audience tries to shush her and explain it's just a play. She in turn shushes them and yells, ever determined: It couldn't hoit! I think this is mildly funny, even though it showcases the immigrant mother's failure to assimilate into middle-class life.) I do not believe that there's a relationship between others praying for you and healing; last year a $2.4 million study concluded the same thing. If you're praying for yourself, that's another matter, one that has to do with repetition and tradition and comfort and belief.

Linc doesn't know this, but I started reciting the Shema prayer to myself at bedtime several years ago. I'd quit at some point after my childhood. I know that God doesn't exist, but I know the prayer exists and has existed for a long, long time. I suppose I'm an animist for believing that the prayer itself has a soul.

◆ ◆ ◆

The Holter monitor did not find arrhythmia in Linc's heart.

May 16. Cloak of Invisibility

I know that certain people don't and won't recognize me. I don't blame them. My hair was my outstanding feature. Without it, I'm a stranger, invisible. That is the fantasy—that we could disguise ourselves and see what people say about us, or pretend to kill ourselves off and witness the funeral. When I was younger (twenty-nine) and my hair had no hint of gray, I passed myself off as a nineteen-year-old college sophomore and went through the paces of sorority rush for the first time. I wanted to see what it was like. I was being judged, but at a safe distance. I had the power. After two rounds, I was busted, but I didn't confess.

I was a spy one other time. The summer before graduate school I took a part-time marketing job at an architecture firm and worked on a novel the rest of the time. I would call potential clients and say I was doing a survey for OWP Marketing about architecture firms. I'd ask, Do you have a firm that you work with? OWP were the initials of my employers. Sometimes the person on the other end would ask, Who are you working for? I forget how I was supposed to respond. I assume that I was supposed to be as vague as possible and never confess.

In fifth and sixth grades, we also conducted surveys. You would get a friend of yours from another school to call a boy you were interested in. She would say, I'm doing a survey. Please rate these girls as potential girlfriends, A, B or C. Your name would be buried somewhere in the middle. She'd ask him to rate cuteness and personality, too. You'd know the results the minute your friend hung up the phone. And the boy knew that his answers would be made public.

How did we come upon this sophisticated marketing technique at age ten and eleven? I still remember that a certain person rated me high in personality. He hadn't been surveyed on my account, but I was pleased to have the information. Now we all have websites and can count our visitors and can look up the status of our books on Amazon and read our students' evaluations of us. And we can help orchestrate the opinions; I knew a feature writer at a newspaper who wanted to become a critic. Every time she wrote a review, random readers (really, her friends), wrote letters to the editor praising her review. And it worked. She became a reviewer.

Or maybe the letters had nothing to do with her promotion.

Then she got breast cancer and it came back and in 2002 she died.

May 19. Free Dinners & Free Dinners

I had a lovely free dinner last night with professors, all writers. The menu was prix fixe so you felt the obligation to order dessert. I did. We all did. I could have ordered more lightly, but there was much butter butter everywhere. My appetizer was two crab cakes with avocado chunks and skinny potato strings. Then I had acorn squash stuffed with risotto. Then sorbet. For some restaurants, butter is the new butter. After I went to bed I got back up and threw up. I'm lucky that the chemo hasn't made me nauseated but it has mangled my digestive system. I was so afraid of nausea, because it's ever constant. So this is better than nausea. But I have to watch myself.

The soup of the day was cream of fennel. It was served with a tall pat of butter in the middle of a bare bowl. Then the soup was poured over it.

This defiantly lavish use of butter—I know it's defiant because we all know about animal fats and cholesterol and good fats and bad fats—is a reaction to the self-satisfied substitution of olive oil. Back to butter. Retro-smug. Retro-rebellious.

My subsidized dinner was with Smart U Day School folks and a lovely, lyrical visiting writer. I am with the Night School. The difference between Day and Night is the difference between... night and day. You saw that one coming. The Day School people, mostly, have full-time contracts. The Night School people are all part time. As I told a prospective student yesterday who wanted to meet me during office hours, I don't have an office. I wrote this to him on e-mail. He wrote back: That sure cuts down on office hours.

Though this isn't to say that the Day School people never teach at night. They do. Then they are Day people moonlighting.

The Day people can be tenured. The Night people are always hanging. *Tenured*, from the verb to hold. We are slippery, we Night people. We slither, frictionless, through the groves of academe. We can break bread with the Day people, we can partake of their largesse, and then we slink our way to another institution and then back, as if we know where we're going.

May 21. The Erotic Life of Property

I went to a funeral today, my third in the past year. In Jewish lore, you are performing a good deed to put a shovelful of earth on the coffin, because that person can never repay you. I didn't know that you were supposed to stick the shovel back in the pile of dirt and not hand it to the next person. The reason, the rabbi told us, is because we are supposed to be reluctant in performing this task, reluctant to bury this person who was just among us. I didn't know the person who died. I knew his son Cory (my student) and daughter-in-law, and had met his ex-wife. When I'd told Cory that I had cancer, he said something like it feeling like I was family. He'd been in two of my classes and I'd supervised his internship. His family had sent me flowers, so going to the funeral seemed to be the thing to do, to continue this circle of participating in important events in each other's lives.

For many years I did not understand why my parents' friends—people I didn't know—had sent me presents on my bat mitzvah. I figured it out when I read *The Gift: Imagination and the Erotic Life of Property* by Lewis Hyde. He talks about how gifts define community. Then I was able to see that the bat mitzvah gift was more than one gift, it was a gesture in a (then-)35-year chain of gestures and connections. I still have a letter that one of my father's friends wrote me on my bat mitzvah. It was about the friendship of our families. That man recently died and my mother went to the funeral and then to the shiva. Here, I have the letter, in my Nonfiction files, under the man's last name. He wrote: *Your father and I went to school together and have remained close friends over the years. Unfortunately we (you and I) have not gotten to know each other as well as I would have liked. It is not unusual in this busy fast moving world of ours for good friends to see little of one another in comparison to the time spent together as children and young adults. As each takes on additional responsibilities, less time is available for "get togethers." You will discover this when you get older. Then you will realize that a great many of your friends remain close to you even though you do not see them as often as you would like.*

He wrote to me as an equal. He thanked me for including his family in the bat mitzvah and after-party. I had nothing to do with his invitation. My parents invited their friends and our relatives, and I invited my friends.

The thing is, despite all the proclaimed warmth of his letter, his family didn't invite my family to many events.

May 23. The Blessing

My accountant asked if cancer changed me. I suppose, slightly. I know more about cancer. I feel more comfortable with people who have it or have had it. I take cabs more often. I don't feel deeper or more grateful or spiritual. She asked if I believed in God more. She was assuming that I believed in God some. No, I told her. Although I have returned, mostly because I have more free time, to Torah study. We're all irreverent and don't believe that the Torah is the divine word. We meet in a science conference room in the nearby Catholic university. Today Stan, a biology professor, told this story:

The other day he'd been in his office when a man stopped at the open door and asked if he was a *kohain*, a member of the priestly class. Stan's last name is Cohn, a variant of Cohen and his name was on the door. (In Judaism, we assume that people named Cohen and the like are descendants of the temple priests.) Stan told him yes, he was a kohain. The other man was very religious, with *tzitzit* (fringes) hanging under his shirt. He was a buyer-back of textbooks; that's why he was roaming the university hallways at this time of year. The man asked if Stan would give him the priestly blessing. Stan is not ritually observant, though he belongs to a progressive synagogue. He never wears a yarmulke (skull cap) but that day—*that day only*—he had one in his pocket because of something having to do with his wife, his car and his glove compartment—one of those explanations that takes too long to delve into. He had the aplomb to whip out the yarmulke from his pocket nonchalantly, and put it on his head. He'd never been asked to bless anyone before, but he happened to know the priestly blessing. He said he knew it from going to services, and had recited the first line of it to bless his daughter when he dropped her off at college. So the religious textbook man was blessed, he thanked the prof, and that was it.

Technically, my husband Linc is a kohain, though he is a true atheist who says of organized religion, *Nisht fur mir* (Not for me.) A couple of years ago he came with me to a family bar mitzvah, where he met my religious young cousin. The cousin was excited to learn that Linc was a kohain and told him that he, Linc, cannot ever become extremely drunk because the messiah could come at any time and Linc would be needed at the synagogue within twenty minutes. I mentioned this at Torah study and the question raised was, Is the twenty minutes so that he can round up an animal to sacrifice? The only handy animal around here is squirrel, and that's not one of the official sacrificial mammals mentioned in the Torah. I know that from my study. Today is the first day of the holiday Shavuos. We should stay up all night studying Torah and eating blintzes, which are thin cheese- or cherry-filled crepes. When I lived in Iowa City I planned a big Shavuos gathering. I called the local supermarket looking for frozen blintzes, which are traditionally served on the holiday. The guy thought it was an obscene phone call. I ended up making them from scratch.

May 27. Post-Funeral

Friday I stopped by the home of a colleague of Linc's. Her mother had died; the service was private, but her home was open for what we call shiva but others might call an open house. I have a memorial service to go to on Tuesday, for the parent of another colleague of Linc's.

A month or so a student gave me a bouquet for helping him with his thesis. One stem of orchids had survived all this time, two fuchsia-and-white dendrobium orchids, open flowers at the bottom, buds at the top. My mother-in-law told me that if you spray the buds with water they'll blossom. I tried it and it's true. The top ones have opened. Now, I hate when people make analogies between Nature and Life, but here I am about to do it myself: The bottom flowers are like an earlier generation. By the time they die out, the new flowers are out and they have no knowledge or relationship (OK, add anthropomorphizing to my list of sins) to the older flowers, so they are not saddened by their demise. OK, this is the way I've thought of it: Ashkenazi Jews name their babies after relatives who have died. I'm named for my grandfather. I feel no sadness about his death, because it preceded me. I remember once in grade school trying not to laugh at something, biting the insides of my cheeks and trying to think of something sad: the death of my grandfather. But it wasn't sad because I hadn't experienced the loss. That is my simple point. And you turn the loss into a gain when you use the name for a new person. Turning sadness to joy. I should see birth as a wondrous thing but all I see when I look at an infant is a lot of trouble. Time, trouble, sleepless nights. That's why I don't have children. And someday my name will go to a relative who isn't here yet. A child named Cancer Bitch.

May 30. Hunting and Gathering

Today at Torah study we were reading that Jews are allowed to eat deer and gazelle, but not sacrifice them.

Gazelle, said Stan, that's the original Jewish fast food.

June 2. Louts

I got off the L yesterday afternoon after the Cubs game let out and the neighborhood was littered, as usual, with drunken and drunken-seeming louts. I was walking behind some on the sidewalk and then in front of them. I could hear them talking about the message on my head: US Out of Iraq. Oh, said one, I gotta put my glasses on to read that. Out? Pull out? That's what my girlfriend says. I can't pull out. We gotta stay in there. We gotta really go in there with soldiers and stay. We can't pull out. We gotta push.
Etc., etc.
When I walked inside my gate and went up the porch steps. I turned and waved.
Later I went with Barry to see a Brecht play up the street. Because he's in a scooter we were on the first row. The theater was small and almost packed, it was the second night, with at least one big critic there. The play was loud and intense, much screaming. Cartoonish. Polemical. Typical Brecht. Some good acting. Finally it ended. We went out. In the little lobby the Big Critic was talking to some people. On the sidewalk there were about fifteen people smoking, including at least one of the actors. There was a static-ness, not a rush to leave.
About two hours later, reading about the play on the Internet, I realized there were scenes we didn't see. We'd left at halftime. Both Barry and I see live theater at least every other month. Between us we must have seen thousands of performances. And there hadn't been a curtain call, after all. But with B's spaciness from his MS and with my chemo brain, we missed the obvious. We were louts.

June 7. Marks

Monday night I talked on the phone to Jodi, my actor friend in Madison, who reported on her performance at a benefit to raise money to build a Gilda's Club there. She used me for source material. She had one of her personas tell the crowd that she had a friend who'd hennaed her head to say Obama in '08. She explained to me that Out of Iraq would be too political. You'd think that all of Madison would be against the war, but Jodi knows her audience. It's a sign of progress that supporting a liberal biracial man for president is considered non-controversial in Madison. But what does it say about the chances for this war to end?

I was standing in line at Emerald City a while ago when one of the other denizens, a cop, asked me why my message didn't say, Support Your Local Police. I demurred: Too many words. He has thick gray hair with a receding hairline. He said that his scalp has a tattoo that says, US Marine Corps. He was young and drunk at the time. How odd to think that his history will be revealed, slowly, if he goes bald, his own personal archaeology.

June 10. **Lump**

My internist had felt a lump in my (former) left breast in August and told me then to get an ultrasound, but since the last time she'd sent me for an ultrasound, the radiologist had found nothing and moreover had pooh-poohed internists as alarmists, I didn't do anything. I had an appointment with my Boyish Gyne soon after and asked him to examine the lump. He said it didn't feel like cancer. Today I had an appointment with him today to check out my fibroids. I had imagined making a dramatic announcement: Remember that lump you said was nothing? Well (whipping open the hospital gown and letting the silence be eloquent)—. He walked in with the motto on his lips of All Doctors Who Know You Have Cancer: Are you hanging in there? It's quite apt but gets tiresome. He did an endometrial biopsy just to make sure there wasn't another cause of my bleeding, such as endometrial dysplasia, a pre-cancerous condition. I didn't have the guts to say, Are you sorry you missed the lump? But I did make reference to the lump, and later he said he was sorry I had cancer.

What did I expect? I had asked him to feel it, as an afterthought, and I hadn't followed my internist's instructions. When I told this to the surgeon she had reassured me that a few months wouldn't have made a difference, that this was slow-growing cancer. The real culprit, if there is one, is the Mammogram Factory, the place where I used to get mammograms, which hadn't picked up the tumor until this year. Or me, for not noticing changes in my breast. But my breasts have been so lumpy and dense and confusing in their lumpiness and density, terra incognita, times two.

June 12. Bleed Me a River

The Boyish Gyne called to say that my biopsies were negative. He hypothesized that I'm in menopause but bleeding because of the fibroids. I don't agree. I think I still have real periods but they're very very looooonnng because of the fibroids. Why would I think this? Am I loath to give up this sign of young womanhood? Maybe. Am I scared? I think I'm scared. Of what, besides death and old age and turning into a crone, a word that feminists reclaimed twenty years ago, after all? Have I enjoyed the sheer weirdness of thirty-eight years of bleeding? The blood seems alive, a sign of life, though I know it's a sign of death (no zygote forming). I am so full of life that I have blood to spare.

Menopause is supposed to cause the fibroids to shrink. But if I'm in menopause already, and am having faux periods caused by fibroids, then it means that menopause is not causing the fibroids to wither, as Engels said the state would, after the proletariat seized the means of production and abolished social classes.

June 13. Guilt

The beginning of this guilt. First a feeling of difference, of feeling what I have isn't serious, not the real thing, starting from reading blogs by people with what they call *mets*—meaning the breast cancer has metastasized. Reading reviews of books by these people—feeling I haven't really had cancer until it's moved from the breast to crack my spine. That it's only, in the words of one blogger, garden variety cancer.

Sunday I heard that an out-of-town acquaintance/friend had had a mastectomy and was having a hard time. I e-mailed her. She e-mailed back. She seemed reticent. I named my meds. She said she was on pretty much the same, and that the experience had been very difficult. I felt guilty that side effects weren't wiping me out. Though I get days in a row when I'm tired and depressed. But now I feel fine. When I feel fine I stop feeling sorry for myself. I feel guilty.

Linc reminded me that I'm not taking Cytoxan, which is one element of the usual so-called ACT chemo brew—Adriamycin, Cytoxan, Taxol—because of my platelet disorder. Cytoxan could cause a blood clot, which is more dangerous than the cancer. It could be the Cytoxan that's causing my friend's side effects. Linc also reminds me that I'm getting less anti-cancer protection, too. I'm lucky that the anesthesia didn't make me sick. My cousin (by marriage) in Marin County was diagnosed just after I was and she threw up for days from the anesthesia as well as the sedative they gave her when they installed her port.

I feel I should be suffering more, that I'm faking it. That I don't really have cancer. That I'm not really getting chemo. How can I be thinking this? Is this a manifestation of denial? No, it's a transmogrification of the essential feeling: that I do not deserve to live. That I should perish soon. I was not made to live a long time. I was made to live tragically. Different from other people. I was made to be mourned. And to mourn while I was alive. Because I did not deserve to be alive. So living was treacherous. I had to live secretly, secretively. Under the radar. Feeling like this because of asthma. Or for no reason I can find.

Let me try to find logic in this feeling about my cancer, here and now. That I feel guilty because I feel good even though I'm supposed to be dying? That seems like it. The Cancer Bitch who would not die even though it was in the cards. She shuffled the deck. Used sleight of hand to change her fate. And then cried out: I am alive, please forgive me.

June 19. The Tongue,

said the endodontist this morning, is a very curious animal. He is working on a root canal that couldn't be postponed. He told me his brother is an oncologist who had cancer in his tonsils and directed his own treatment.

The cancer cell has its compulsions and obsessions. We are told: Normal cells stop dividing when they come into contact with like cells, a mechanism known as contact inhibition. Cancerous cells lose this ability. The cancer cell does not get the social cues. It cannot read the faces of the other cells. It does not know when to stop reproducing itself, when to stop telling that story one more time about its cross-country trip in a beat-up station wagon. Because of this we need to ingest poison to stop the cancer cells, and in so doing, the toxin stops other harmless and helpful cells in their tracks. The faster the cells are dividing, the more likely it is that chemotherapy will kill the cells, causing the tumor to shrink. They also induce cell suicide (self-death or apoptosis).

Cancer cells are uninhibited. They put lampshades on their heads and run through public fountains. But these same frolicking, out-of-control cancer cells are trying to kill us. In defense, we try to induce suicide. Can you blame us?

Today was chemo Round 5, the first dose of Taxol, which is derived from the Pacific yew. We have some kind of yew bushes out front, which we prune. I don't know what kind they are. Taxol is diluted with a castor-oil-based concoction called Cremophor El, which a few people are allergic to. The nurses told me that a reaction is rare, but they laid out epinephrine and Benadryl on the table nearby just in case. They'd already given me some Benadryl in the drip. Reactions include feeling very hot or having constricted breathing. It happens in the first few minutes.

After a few minutes on the drip I felt blood rush to my head and ears and they were hot hot hot, and I felt an invisible heavy foot on my chest and it was hard to breathe. I reported this calmly because they'd said they were prepared. They took me off the Taxol and gave me more Benadryl and put an oxygen cannula in my nostrils. I felt better. Then a few minutes later I had what felt like menstrual cramps, and a nurse gave me a heat pack. The cramps went away in about ten minutes.

Was this anaphylactic shock? I asked. No, said the nurse, it was anaphylaxis. It sounded like the same thing to my untutored ears.

My mother had come to town for my chemo, and remained perfectly calm, too. It was all because the nurses said they were prepared.

June 24. Taking Taxol/I feel petty, oh, so petty

What can I say about chemotherapy that hasn't already been said, in a million pop songs? That's a line from an essay by TV writer Marjorie Gross. I don't know what chemo-poison she was referring to. (She died of ovarian cancer.) The chemotherapy agent of the hour, of my hour of discontent, is Taxol. Sounds like *toxic*. It seems like toxic. A drug that's injected in your veins that makes your bones hurt. Not like when you were little and your mother would mention offhand to your doctor you felt *growing pains*. No, this is an ache in the joints and along the bones, that seems maybe it's not so bad, it's not acute, but it's there. Deep and unrelieved, and it makes you cry during yoga when you bury your head for Child's Pose. Because it doesn't seem like it should hurt so much. And you cry partly because you suspect you're exaggerating the hurt, and partly because of the hurt itself. The pain is real, it's from the wiping out of red blood cells, and it's there in the pink oncology binder, in black and white, under Side Effects. And the nurse told you it might happen. It's the subtlety of it, as cruel as mean girl gossip, almost not there, but there. And in your teeth, making them feel loose, and in your gums and a sharp sore on the side of your tongue, and an ache in your back, and you feel it in your endometrium, like a bad cramp, though there aren't bones there.

◆ ◆ ◆

Friday after yoga I drove downtown to pick up Linc so we could meet Val for dinner in the South Loop. When he got in the car to take my place (I hate driving) I was crying and we pulled to the corner and I told him I felt so bad. He took me home and called V to cancel. I was so pathetic, so grateful that he was driving me home. We stopped at Blockbuster and got four DVDs: *Curb Your Enthusiasm*, first season; *Sex and the City*, second season; *The Truth About Cats and Dogs* and *Sweet Home Alabama*. At home I settled on the couch and he unloaded the dishwasher and did other household chores while I watched *Sex and the City*, which he can't stand but gets sucked into anyway. I took acetaminophen, which he said I should have been taking instead of ibuprofen. And lo and behold, it was the pain-reliever of choice in the pink oncology department binder from Fancy Hospital. I felt better and also whiny and self-indulgent.

Now it's Sunday evening and what I've done this weekend is Nothing, meaning watched the videos and read some and slept. And wrote a pissy letter to the editor about the whitewashing of

Nicaraguan history in the Travel section of the paper. I did what dogs do, which is lie around and nap and then get up and sleep. If dogs read, I'd be the perfect dog. Linc has told me that I'm silly to feel guilty for doing nothing, aka Taking Care of Myself. I was invited to a barbecue, which I skipped, and was supposed to go to a Muslim festival to help publicize a Muslim-Jewish poetry anthology I'm helping put together. You have cancer! he tells me, and I say, Supposedly the cancer is gone, but he counters that I'm going through cancer treatment, and what I'm feeling is because of that treatment. Which is true. The bone pain has lessened much, and I'm wondering if what I felt is what it's like when the cancer returns and it's in your bones.

♦   ♦   ♦

Last night I dreamed I looked for my mailbox in the Smart U journalism department and couldn't find it. In real life, a number of years ago, my faculty mailbox disappeared from the journalism department. The mailbox itself didn't disappear—the label with my name on it did. The reason was I had started teaching non-credit instead of credit journalism classes, and the Decider of Mail Boxes had decided I didn't deserve a box. Though there were lots of empty boxes. I eventually got hold of an empty cardboard box and put it on top of the mail boxes, with my name on it. The whole box was taken away and then I got another box and labeled it ETAOIN SHRDLU, which is an old journalism (nonsense) phrase from the days of Linotype. It's made up of the dozen most common letters in English. I told a good friend about all this a few years later and he told me how terrible I was to have done this. He used the word asshole, which was the first and only time anyone has called me that, at least to my face. When he said that I felt I'd been petty and immature. It is unwise in academia to be petty and immature unless you have tenure.

I still have a mailbox problem. I'm a part-time, year-round employee at Smart U but my mailbox downtown is removed during the quarters I'm not teaching on that campus. I have tried repeatedly to change this, but the person who makes and inserts the mail box labels goes by a book of faculty names she gets every quarter and that's that. The assistant dean tried to intervene once but he couldn't get me a box. Sometimes I make my own mailbox label and feel like an illegal squatter and wonder if the mail sorters will ignore it because the label isn't like the others.

This non-box-ness makes me feel disappeared. I try not to think about it. Until I had these real estate crises, I used to think the comic strip *Dilbert* was ridiculous and unrealistic.

July 4. Taxol: Once More, with Feeling

I had my second round or session or infusion of Taxol on Monday, with chemo escort Sharon. When I told the warm and helpful Nurse Lora about the bone pain, she asked what number it was from 1-10. I said 3, but that I felt like crying. She laughed and said it sounded more like 10, and she wrote me a prescription for a short-term corticosteroid (dexamethasone), to take prophylactically.

Last night was the first July 3 Linc and I have spent together in Chicago without going downtown for the fireworks. Linc thought that being surrounded by a million people wouldn't be the best thing for a Cancer Bitch with a depressed immune system. We rode bikes, looking at houses and condos we pretended to ourselves we were interested in, then went to a new branch of a Mexican restaurant around the corner, even though we'd bought all kinds of organic produce Monday night. The guacamole was good, the chips were oily. At home, we spent about ten minutes on the roof looking at the top edges of the fireworks behind the Hancock Building. The rain drove us in. In the middle of the night I threw up.

I woke up this morning with slight joint pain, took the steroid and went back to sleep. Now the pain or discomfort is gone. That's the $64,000 question: What is the line between pain and discomfort?

July 8. Pain & Pain

The topic for today is pain and pain—pain that causes weeping and pain that comes with weeping, and how difficult it is to tell the difference between the two. After my first Taxol infusion, I had joint and bone pain that made me cry three days later. So I sat around and watched DVDs and TV for two days. This time around, I came armed with a corticosteroid to stave off the pain. Nurse Linc told me it could cause anxiety, so take it morning and mid-afternoon, not evening. And then on the third day after the second Taxol, I was anxious, terribly anxious, because of the drug, because I was writing a book review and I'm not wired to write book reviews, they make me anxious, they tax a part of the brain I don't have. And the fourth day, I was in some joint pain, not too much, but felt like crying. I was anxious and depressed. Desperately depressed. I went to yoga and felt like crying and only sorted it out later that it wasn't because of pain or tiredness but because of depression. Soul-corroding depression. The kind of depression where the world seems like a vast desert and there's nothing to connect to, to hold onto, that every human in the universe is just a little desperate bucket of misery searching for distraction. And you can carry on a conversation in the midst of this depression, but the conversation is going on a parallel, pretend-world, what's real is the feeling underneath you can't shake, that nothing matters. And you can't stand it.

And then I would feel sadder and sadder, thinking that this is how I felt in my twenties and thirties, and I'd wonder how many other people are feeling this, all the time. I went through motions, we went to dinner, to a movie, we rode our bikes home, I wrote about this depression, and then in bed I cried and cried and told Linc all this, and he listened and it wasn't much better but we went to sleep.

And in the morning I was OK. I didn't feel the doubleness. I didn't take the last corticosteroid. I felt a little shaky Saturday but I felt like myself. I could laugh. I could connect with the world. My joints hurt a little, and I took a little acetaminophen. I watched some TV, finding myself for the second time this summer watching some show with Dick Van Dyke as a doctor. We rode bikes to dinner with Mitch. We talked about periods of depression. He was impressed that mine went away in a day. But it was still so horrible.

The Taxol caused the weeping. The corticosteroid caused the depression. Next time I'll get help for treating the emotion. I think that's much worse than the pain. But the pain is pain.

July 9. Suffering

If anybody ever offers you the choice between suffering and depression, take the suffering. And I don't mean physical suffering. I mean emotional suffering. I am hereby endorsing psychic suffering over depression.

Don't get me wrong; suffering, though universal, and though its universality provides the basis of Buddhism, is bad. Today I suffered. It meant being weepy, rageful at the drop of a pin, filled with ire at someone for being fourteen minutes late (when it didn't matter at all; and I didn't show my rage) and at a fucking stupid fucking imbecile waiter at Kopi Café who didn't know that a goddam fucking matte is supposed to be dark and smoky, and not the color and taste of pale green swill with little green specks in it. (I didn't yell. I had a sharpness to my voice a few notches below sarcasm and I smiled deceitfully. I gave a good tip.) Then I went to Women & Children First bookstore down the street and when the clerk asked how I was doing, I said softly, I'm suffering, probably sounding melodramatic but not meaning to. In yoga I wasn't able to balance in Warrior I pose because my toes were numb from the horrible Taxol. I felt like crying, not because of pain, really, but just because I felt like crying. I wept into my purple yoga mat while folded into Child's Pose and then wept face up into the open air with closed eyes and sweaty head while lying on my back with my legs in butterfly and then I accepted defeat, that the weeping would not end, and rolled up said mat and walked up the street to the drugstore to pick up some refills and a drug that Nurse Lora had just called in to combat the numbness. Suffering was going to the drug store and finding out that the very new dolt of a clerk didn't have my new drug, it would take ten minutes, he said. I was weeping and hovering at the counter like a desperate addict in my rain-dropped-on bald head, T-shirt and torn shorts, and I went back to him and said, Could you give me just a pill or two for now, and finally, Could you make a little faster because I'm in a lot of pain, and I felt a little guilty because I wasn't in pain-pain, not about-to-die-and-double-over pain, but in weepiness pain, the pain of not wanting to be there, standing around and weeping and feeling a hole in my heart of desperation and sadness and rage. A dark wound in my heart. And suffering meant walking home with my three drugs finally, my umbrella above my head, knowing I would be home soon, where I would be able to collapse and even work on the stupid idiotic fucking book review, because I was suffering and not depressed. Suffering meant I knew that crying would make me feel better, once I could stop, and that I knew that underneath the suffering I had a core of appreciation for the thunderstorm that had broken the hot spell this afternoon, even though it had drenched my poor bike and helmet that I'd left moored to a parking meter on the street. Underneath the suffering was psychic pain, which is an entity, but I can deal with an entity, it is better than the erosion created by depression, which is more absent than absence, depression is the oxygen-gulping aridness of the void, and it fills every part of you with the knowledge that nothing matters, the universe is as meaningless as it is infinite. So that there is no part of you left that can slither its way around and get its interest quickened by an idea or person or mind or glazed blue Moroccan tile. There is no room for beauty or Marx or charity or alternatives to war. There is only the ash that's left after a fire, after a long, long rain.

July 13. The Dancer's Pose

At yoga we often do partner work. One day last week we paired up to help one another do Dancer's Pose. My partner was one of The Twins in the Back. The Twins are girls who look about twenty and have dark, wavy hair. Usually they partner with one another. You can't blame them; they're perfectly matched by height and weight. Lately they've come with a third girl who's shorter. I'd said hello to them but never talked to them before. They always stay on the back row, in a corner. This time only one of them was in class. She asked me about my head tattoo and I told her I was going through chemo. She said that she went through chemo *in my country*. She's from Peru, it turns out, and she was diagnosed with lymphoma at fourteen. She had chemo and radiation for two years. It was in Lima, and she lived about a mile from the hospital. She said her family was really close, that there are four girls. She also said it was very hard to lose her hair at fourteen. It makes you stronger, she said.

Today in class all three were there, and all in the back. I did partner work with Garnett. I wanted to at least catch the eye of the twin I talked to last week. But I couldn't tell which one she was.

July 16. Chemo Day

Garnett picked me up and took me to Fancy for my noon chemo appointment. She had to leave at 3:30 and passed the baton to Linc. At one point I asked him to get me a blanket because I was cold, but by the time he found one, I'd had a hot flash and was sweating. As I told Lora, the hot flashes are the least of my problems. Feeling the void in the world is the worst, followed closely by bone pain and then weeping mixed with irritability.

Yesterday my friend Jennifer was in town from Ohio, and we had brunch with her hosted by Rabbi Roy, who married us at the Bourgeois Pig, and his wife Frida. Jennifer graciously decorated my scrubbed and shaved head with curlicues, filigree, tiny peace signs and grape leaves and an easy-to-read US out of Iraq in back. My head was quite the hit in Chemolandia today. Jennifer is a professional artist and did a lovely job. Some of it is jagua, a black fruit-based ink. Most of it is henna, which is a greenish paste that dries black and eventually peels or falls off to reveal red-brown underneath. I try to keep the dark on as long as possible but it's so tempting to peel and pick. It's like fifth grade when everyone was pouring glue on their palms and pulling off the dried "skin." It's as satisfying as stomping on plastic bubble wrap. Not everybody appreciates that pleasant activity. Which is too bad.

July 23. The Million-Dollar Brazilian

Well, first of all, it's probably not a million dollars. It's probably going to add up to $100,000, billed to insurance. But the *hundred-thousand-dollar Brazilian* just doesn't cut it. Doesn't begin to conjure up that sexy gal from Ipanema. What I'm talking about is the outrageous and barbaric practice of paying someone to apply hot wax to your pubic hair and rip it out. I don't know anybody who's had this done. Or rather, nobody's told me she's had this done. Probably I know lots of women, young women, very young women, who have undergone this procedure. I just haven't seen the evidence. According to an *Esquire-Marie Claire* survey last fall, 66 percent of women in their twenties have their pubic hair trimmed or waxed, and 18 percent keep it bare. Half of women in their forties have their hair trimmed or waxed, and only 5 percent have it bare. Or *clean*, as some put it. A Brazilian, according to articles I've read, is either having every bit of hair yanked out, or leaving a *landing strip* or *Hitler's mustache*. The practice is outlawed in the UK, which seems wise—so that a celebrity I've never heard of, who's the widow of someone else I've never heard of, jets from England to J. Sisters International Salon in New York to be waxed by one of the seven Brazilian sisters who should have been arrested at the border for importing this practice.

In *Shape* magazine I saw a full-page ad I didn't quite understand, but slowly figured out was for a product that allowed you to wax your pubic hair into various shapes. The question is: Why? Beyond a passing attack of whimsy? Apparently, *Shape* readers are used to waxing themselves and it didn't have to be spelled out. According to feminist Naomi Wolf, heterosexual men want women to be bare because they want their sex partners to look like porn stars.

Cancer Bitch has never waxed anything, including floors and furniture, though in her youth she bleached her mustache and arm hairs. Now she doesn't have to because Adriamycin and Taxol have left her hair-depleted. She has two half-eyebrows, just a little hair left on her shins, and a threadbare little nest above her crotch. How can I say this delicately? There's a slit underneath the nest. It reminds her of the profile of a crocodile. The slit was covered for years and she forgot it was there. Forgot that her self was shaped like that, in front. In fact, Cancer Bitch saw a painting in the Uffizi Gallery that showed just such a slit and she thought the painter had erred. She's surprised to see herself like this in the mirror. Her skin feels soft, very soft, velvety in fact, but all wrong.

Cancer Bitch has wanted to discuss this topic for a while, but has been afraid. She is non-tenured and non-tenure-track. About fifteen years ago a colleague, who was an inspiration to the rest of the adjuncts because he had finagled a year-long contract that included health insurance, lost it all with just a few words. He appeared on TV with his girlfriend, either naked or having sex or both. Probably the images were blurry. The appearance included an interview, in which he mentioned, unfortunately, where he taught. Alumni from the department were upset and made it known. And soon there was no more lucky colleague with a contract and health insurance at Smart University. There were few traces of him, either, except here and there in a file drawer were some photocopies with his name on it.

I'm afraid that the president of Smart U will read this...and what? Is Cancer Bitch puffed up with her own importance? She's insulting the president by imagining him to be narrow-minded. And after all, this is why the second wave of feminists fought, so that in the early 21st century, a Cancer Bitch could write about her loss of pubic hair with impunity.

July 25. Barry-watch

Barry spent last night on the floor next to his bed. His helper didn't show up last night and his cellphone was downstairs. The helper showed up this morning and got him dressed and into his scooter. Barry called me to come and plug in his new scooter. It took both of us about twenty minutes to figure out where on the scooter you plug in the plug-thing. I couldn't read the info booklet without my reading glasses, and Barry said it didn't tell you where the cord went. But as I said, finally we prevailed. You'd think that a manufacturer of scooters for disabled people would have a special easy way to recharge the battery of the thing.

July 30. I Hate Fancy Hospital

It is 11:30 am and I should be on my way to my last chemo appointment, along with my friend Sylvienne who flew in from San Francisco for escort duty, but Fancy does not have me on the schedule. In fact, I am not on the schedule until a month hence. I called this morning to see if I needed to be there at noon, my appointment time, or later, because I often wait and wait in the huge and distressing cancer ward waiting area. I also called because I remembered I didn't get a printout of this appointment, though it was understood I was coming in today at noon. Or I thought it was understood. After seven sessions on Mondays at noon (one on a Tuesday because of a holiday), and being told that Taxol is administered every two weeks, I thought it was obvious that I should be seen today at noon. But my nurse is on vacation, and I think her backup is on vacation, and given Fancy Hospital's tendency to overbook (Worse than the airlines? I can't decide) I should not assume anything. But I did. I am very very very upset.

My voice cracks when I talk on the phone to the receptionists and chemo administrative director and the nurse who called me back after she was paged twice in 45 minutes. And so now it is 11:52 and I have been called back and told I have my appointment at 1:00 pm. I can't tell you how momentous the last day of chemo is. It is, well, the last day of chemo. The end of the beginning. The end of feeling you are blasting the cancer away and now you are left up to your own devices and Tamoxifen.

◆ ◆ ◆

When I got to Fancy the receptionist said that I had missed my appointment with the oncologist—which no one had been aware of when I spoke to staff on the phone. The doctor came around during chemo, and neither he nor his assistant apologized for the screw-up. And then chemo was over.

My mother says that at M.D. Anderson the nurses ring a little bell to signal someone's end of chemo. Would it kill the people at Fancy to do *something* in commemoration?

August 1. Quaver

I woke up today without a quaver in my voice or in my chest. Yesterday I could feel the quaver, the tears, as a liquid entity, filling ligaments or pipelines, or something, across my chest. Like they were there, an unending supply, and it wouldn't do any good to cry them out because there would be more. I could talk but if it was about anything remotely personal (how do I feel, what am I thinking) I was weepy weepy weepy, weeping. Sylvienne from San Francisco and I went to Thousand Waves Spa yesterday to get massages. Mine was free as part of the spa's lovely Stress Management Program for women with cancer. She paid retail for hers, and she paid for my massage therapist's tip, as well. We were going to go to Gilda's Club next for a new member orientation, but I felt I couldn't deal with it. Meaning I couldn't imagine sitting around and talking to people. I called to cancel. When I'd called to enroll earlier in the day, the intake person asked why I was interested, and I said I was desperate. When I canceled I was still desperate, even more so.

We went to Dairy Queen then came home and watched *Breakfast at Tiffany's*, which was very different from the way both of us had remembered it. Holly Golightly's less waif and more gold digger. Mickey Rooney is cast, disturbingly, as a Gnashing Oriental neighbor. The role is stereotypical and crass.

When Linc came home we made a tray of whole grain bread, cheese, fruit, hummus and olive tapenade and watched *But I'm a Cheerleader*, a very light movie about a high school cheerleader who's not hetero enough for her Christian parents and her friends, so is sent away to rehab for straightening. Of course she emerges with a lover. Happily, her parents accept her back. I was in the mood for light movies.

Still I was weepy. My sister called and I told her how weepy I was and she said that I had been so strong before. Everyone has the impression that I've been Strong and Courageous. But I don't know what means. I just hadn't been weepy much before.

Audrey Hepburn was English-Dutch, born in Brussels. Her English father walked out on the family. Both parents were Nazi sympathizers, but after her mother moved the family to the Netherlands, and saw her native land invaded, the mother soon supported the Resistance. According to some accounts, Hepburn saw the execution of her uncle for his Resistance work, and saw Jews killed in the street. She studied ballet and performed in concerts to raise money for the Resistance, and was also a courier. During the famine toward the end of the war, she suffered with the rest of the population, subsisting on tulip bulbs and grasses. This may have affected her metabolism.

Except when she was pregnant, she kept herself down to 103 pounds. She was five-foot-seven. In 1987 she became the UNICEF goodwill ambassador, and died in 1993 at age sixty-three of colon cancer, by some accounts, but it may have been cancer of the appendix.

Hepburn was allegedly offered the title role in *The Diary of Anne Frank*, but refused because she was afraid it would stir up too much internal trauma.

August 7. The Never-Ending End

This morning I was on my way to meet a creative-writing client at Emerald City when a young man on a bicycle asked me for directions. I told him how to get to where he was going, and then he asked me about the message on my head. You must feel really strongly, he said. I felt unmasked. My head as canvas was a side effect, not a deliberate political act. I told him that I lost my hair from chemo. I started to feel that if I were really committed, I would have shaved my head back when I had hair. But I guess a button will have to do when the hair sprouts back.

I had to go today to Fancy Hospital to get blood tests before I can get my port removed. Then I went down to the fourth floor for an MRI of the remaining breast. I went by myself and it felt routine. Ah, I remember just a few months ago when an MRI was a big deal. Before I went inside the machine, the tech needed to mark the places on my breast where I had scars, and she used vitamin E capsules to do it. She just taped the golden ovals onto my breast. She said the vitamin E shines up brightly in the pictures. I asked her who thought of that. She didn't know.

Afterwards, I went to Smart U to photocopy some handouts. I saw Hugo there, who mans the desk in the hallway. I told him I was through with chemo. So you're in remission? he asked. I guess, I said. The word scares me because Jesse was in remission. And then his cancer came back.

I stopped in at Barry's tonight. He was in the midst of moving himself from one mechanized wheelchair to another. He fell. It took quite a while to get him from the floor to the sofa. He can move his arms and hands but he doesn't have much strength in them. His legs are dead weights. He told me that the Irregular Helper had called to say she couldn't come tonight. I said, I'm not going to help you get ready for bed. I keep telling him he has to hire someone better. He says a reliable service is too expensive. I figure if we don't help he'll be forced to hire someone else. Linc came over and we moved Barry to the chair. I relented and we were going to help Barry go to bed but he wasn't ready. He wanted to watch Jon Stewart. So we didn't. We shall hope for the best.

He has the kind of MS that just gets worse and worse. There is no remission. Sharon has put him on some supplements, which seems to make him more alert. The doctor says the disease is eating up his spine. He has pain and spasms and his legs shake. I said, You still get pleasure from life, don't you? He said he does sometimes. He said when he wakes up in the morning he doesn't hate the fact that he's still alive.

I will get the results from the MRI in a few days. I need to remember that there are often false positives with the MRI. That's the origin of two of the scars: core biopsies taken earlier this year, which proved to be negative for cancer.

August 13. Port Removal Authority

Friday I got the port removed. It was a fairly simple process, but beforehand I had to go through blood testing, as mentioned, and much bureaucracy.

While I was waiting for the port removal I started talking to three older women—two friends who had come with a third who had to get her new port looked at. I asked how long she was going to have chemo and she said, The rest of my life.

Oh. That kind of breast cancer. The kind that spread.

She'd been cancer-free for six years. She said it was a good six years, that she'd traveled to Europe. When she was going through treatment the first time, she was living with her sister, who had also been diagnosed with breast cancer. Now her sister has cancer in her lungs and adrenal glands. She said she's accepted that if that's what God wants for her, it's OK. She was at peace with dying. Though she didn't say that outright. Her friends were trying to lighten things: Oh, you'll be fine, etc.

But her disease can't be cured, can only be contained at this point.

Friday afternoon a doctor called to report that the MRI results were fine, and that I didn't need to be tested again until next summer. Here's hoping. As Emily Dickinson said, *Hope is the thing with feathers.* I would add, The thing with feathers is the back of a woman I saw in line at the Jewel. Her boyfriend had tattooed the wings on her shoulder blades. She offered me his business card but I traffic only in tattoos that are temporary.

August 24. Damn, Damn, Damn

Grace Paley died yesterday.
Breast cancer.

August 27. Hair is Still MIA

Last night I saw Sharon for the first time since she left for Mexico in July. She asked me if I'd shaved my head; she was expecting that my hair would have returned by now. Alas, I am still hairless. The oncology nurse said that I would keep losing hair three weeks after the last chemo. The last chemo treatment was four weeks ago. Most of my head markings are faded, too, except some messy ones around my face. I am bored with head markings. I am tired of rounding up head-decorators. I am tired of ordering tiny bottles of black jagua ink for $25 a pop, and having the black sludge inside turn runny and difficult after a month.

My attention has turned to the incision where the port was removed. It's a one-and-half-inch horizontal cut between my collarbone and (right) breast. It had super-glue-type stuff on it and a stitch or two, covered by steri-strips. The steri-strips fell off. Linc and I went to Oregon for his birthday in mid-August. The day we left Chicago the incision had scabbed up and had a little pus in it and itched. There was a little pink around the edges. Our first night in Portland we had dinner with two former steelworker pals of Linc's. They're both MDs now. One specializes in infectious diseases and I asked her to look at the cut. She said it looked fine. I asked if I could put antibiotic ointment on it and she said I could if I wanted to. Since, I've had a series of Band-Aids (some with antibiotic on them) and both the cut and the skin around the cut (where the adhesive part of the Band-Aid adhered) have been pink and itchy, so much so that there's a pink square surrounding the cut. We're home now and the cut is bloody and oozy. I have a large, non-latex Band-Aid on it and no antibiotic cream. It doesn't itch. There's no pink around the wound itself, no streaks coming from it, so it's not infected. I think there are two schools of thought when it comes to cuts. One is to let it scab up, but then it leaves a scar. The other is to cover it and keep it moist, and it doesn't scar as much. But I think covering it and putting antibiotic ointment on it may make it, paradoxically, more susceptible to infection. I'm sure I'm displacing all my cancer anxiety on this small cut, but knowing that doesn't keep me from obsessing.

August 28. Night with Barry

Barry phoned when we were just going out the door to buy food. His elevator hasn't been working for a week, and he was stranded outside his building. Sharon's semester has started already, and she was in Indiana, teaching. Their downstairs tenant had carried him and his scooter down earlier so Barry could go out and teach. Now the neighbor was away for the evening at a concert and Barry was at the foot of the porch stairs.

We went over there and first saw the empty scooter. Then we saw legs behind it. He had fallen out and was lying curled up with his head resting on the first step to the porch. We got him sitting up and I brought him some food from upstairs. Meanwhile, I called my mother, who had called earlier. She said we should call the fire department. But they did that last week when his Irregular Helper got stuck in the elevator. The elevator repairman had come today but hadn't succeeded in fixing it, and didn't bother to call Barry to tell him he hadn't fixed it. We were thinking we would sit and wait with him until his tenant came back.

The Cubs had just won against Milwaukee and the lights of Wrigley illuminated the yard for a while. Barry's house is three doors down from the stadium. When the lights went out, Linc pointed to the bats (the mammal) careening around and we watched them fluttering and I could see why people used to think they were birds.

I asked Barry if the Irregular Helper was coming, and he said yes, he expected her between 10:30 and 11:00. I asked if the Helper's brother could come, because he sometimes does. I had never met him but asked if he might be strong enough to carry Barry upstairs. Barry called and about twenty minutes later the cavalry came riding up in a bike. With Linc steadying him, the brother carried Barry up two flights. He and Linc took the scooter apart and carried it upstairs.

And then we came home. I didn't know whether to weep or scream. I didn't do either. When I say to Barry, you have to move, you have to move into a building with multiple elevators, you can find a vintage one like in the converted Wieboldt's department store building by Whole Foods, you can live on one floor instead of two and make everything open and accessible, when I say that, I know I'm saying what I and others have said for over two years, and he knows he's heard me say it millions of times, but he and Sharon have no intention of moving. They love their hundred-year-old frame house with its three sets of staircases and garden (tomatoes, cukes, beans, phlox, peonies, apples). They love the hardwood floors they've had refinished and the walls that Sharon has painted different colors over the years, and they love the two decks above the front porch. They love it all and don't want to leave. They don't want anything to change.

September 8. September Song

That my hair has not returned. That I have about twenty little white hairs scattered all over my scalp, about a half-inch long each. And nothing more. That I visited the dentist twice last week as part of the world's most-protracted root-canal procedure, and the temporary crown has fallen out. That my husband does not feel bad for nagging me. That he nags me because of the weight I gained since I met him, his nagging coming in the form of little unwanted suggestions about exercise. That he would say it's all about exercise. That I cannot control my paperwork. That paper is crowding all around me. That I am mired in yet another book review. That I forget words. That I couldn't think, for instance, of what to call that machine next to the radio, the Cuisinart. That I am a pause-er more than in the past because of this aphasia. That I've had this aphasia and gaps in my memory since I was thirty. That I can't blame it all on chemo-brain. That I am tired. That I am more tired than in the middle of chemo. That people ask, When did they say your hair would be back? But They didn't tell me. That when I ask my friend Miz P about paperwork she tells me she saves every single letter and then reveals that she and her husband lease a storage space. That I tell a non-pack-rat about the invoice from 1982 for my payment as a stand-up comic ($10) and she says, You can't throw that away! That I have gone through this life-changing medical event and have not changed my life. That I can smell fishiness coming from the empty bag of salmon jerky in the trash, the same jerky that jerked out part of my temporary crown. That I am still wrestling with the novel or whatever it is that I started in the summer of 1991. That I read reviews in the paper and I'm jealous or envious of both the reviewer and the author of the book reviewed. That I'm not getting any younger. That I am dying. That a man in my new yoga class looks like my podiatrist, and that young people don't have podiatrists. That my heel hurts when I walk more than a mile despite the new orthotics and the silicone slip-on ankle-thing. That I have to finish the syllabus for class Sept. 18 and was going to print it out to work on it in Emerald City Coffee but I ran out of printer cartridges. That I had to get the air conditioner fixed yesterday. That we have that crack in the bedroom wall. That the mantel looks better without all the cards on it but also looks forlorn and sad. That I feel sad looking at it without its lovely cards bearing good personal wishes for my health and happiness. That my mother can tell on the phone that I'm walking and if I was in that good of shape she shouldn't be able to hear me breathing like that, should she? That my books have outgrown my shelves. That I'm not Grace Paley. That everyone else has more books (that they've written). That I have no discipline. That I have no children, so where has all that time gone? That even people who've had children are so much skinnier than I am. That I have cassette recordings of things I don't care about any more but I don't want to throw away the tapes because it's wasteful but it takes too much time to record emptiness over them. That the pile of scratch paper is too tall. That you can't save everything. That I don't know if I'd regret it if I threw away the receipt of payment for being a standup comic. That I have a box of stories I wrote in graduate school and haven't looked at them in years so why am I saving them? That I miss the cards on the mantel already, including one with woodcuts of cardinals on it from two years ago. That I am such a foolish person that my goose-lamp wears a Cubs outfit I bought for her. That it's September and I haven't sent out any new work to literary magazines. That the 15th is the deadline for a contest of recorded essays and I don't have a clue about the technology involved. That I don't know how many people are coming to dinner on Wednesday. That I haven't called the fish market to order the fish for it or decided whether it will be gumbo or cioppino and which did I have last year or both? That other people don't have six four-drawer file cabinets. That I didn't think I would have to keep ordering henna and fruit-ink from that place in California, almost six weeks after the last chemo treatment. That I plan to change oncologists because the current one seems bored by my case but he's leading a meeting about new treatments in cancer in two weeks and I'm afraid if I change before then he'll be upset when he sees me. That I bother to think that. That in reality he should be bothered by why I wanted to change, should use that as a cue to look inside himself. That really I'm afraid I'll feel embarrassed to see him. That I haven't sent out all the forms for pathology reports that I should, to aid in the genetic counselor's work. That I don't have a schedule or a routine. That I don't have discipline. That I have vitiligo, splotches of skin without pigment. That Barry's sister had it but it went away after she stopped drinking milk. That I think about quitting dairy and then I don't. That I do for a little while and then I don't. That everything makes me weary. That the thought of carrying rice milk with me everywhere makes me weary. That I used to walk longer without getting tired. That I'm not sure what getting tired means. That I don't know if it's the body or the mind, the eyes, the sleepiness of the eyes. That I have hot flashes that melt the ink on my head. That the henna I bought on Devon Avenue faded on my head after two days, after Garnett's lovely design job. That the bicycle seat needs to be raised. That everyone is ahead of me. That I don't know what I really mean but I know it's true. That I have on my desk a blank taxi-cab receipt, a brochure from a Portland restaurant about mindful breathing, a box of bills, my old planner and my new one, two Diet Dr. Pepper cans and so much more. That there is always so much more, including a computer monitor I haven't used in about two years. That I say to myself: If you throw that away, you might regret it, but you can live with the regret. That for months I did sun salutations in the morning and then for months and months I didn't and this morning I did just one Downward-Facing Dog because I was too lazy to unroll the mat. That I slept fourteen-and-a-half hours today, and thus missed both an anti-war demonstration at my congressman's office and a barbecue for Obama. That I'm afraid I'm for Obama only because he's more exciting than Hillary. That I don't care who wins as long as s/he is a Democrat. That I should decide. That I still resent the Obama for Senate campaign for sending us out to register voters without signage and without the capacity to really register them, we were in reality pre-registering them. That the papers are stacked and stacked. That I have four versions of a reading packet from teaching ten years ago. That I know whole families live in houses the size of my office. That I am not mindful. That I don't like the pictures I glued onto the cover of my new calendar-planner. That they seem too chaotic. The central one is of Simon Rodia and Watts Towers. That I was in LA last fall and forgot to go see Watts Towers. That I want to build a Watts Towers. A monument. Something grand and crazy and built bit by bit. To last.

September 11. Rosh Hashanah

Tomorrow is New Year's Eve for Jewish year 5768. I was shocked to read that among the traditional foods eaten on the Jewish new year are black-eyed peas, which I always eat on the first day of the secular new year. So my Texas and Jewish heritages converge. The peas and other foods (such as sheep's head) supposedly arouse the heart to prayer. I am planning to make kosher gumbo, made without shellfish and also without the heads of fish or mammals. The fishmongers at Dirk's will even de-bone and cut up the fish for me.

My mother told me she had to pick up a special security parking card today for her synagogue parking lot in Houston. This is in addition to her parking lot sticker, which was mailed to her. I am going to be taking the L to a little synagogue in Rogers Park on the Far North Side, because Rabbi Roy is no longer leading services at my usual place, the Catholic university down the street. The little synagogue in Rogers Park is invisible. It meets inside a visible church. Just like our congregation met inside a Catholic institution. In a way you could say we're hidden Jews but there are always signs pointing to where we are gathering. And if there are no signs you can just follow the guy on the street holding the velvet tallis bag.

I am reading *Seek My Face: A Jewish Mystical Theology* by Arthur Green. He doesn't talk (so far) about believing in God or not believing in God, but says that the Hebrew word for God is a verb, and that that verb is what's behind growth everywhere. And that we are all part of everything and each other, a notion that we would call Zen. Or physics. I know all this, that we are dust and air, and yet I am so critical of all who are Other. A blond women in pink who is walking too slowly on Michigan Avenue. On the L a pudgy woman with dyed red hair in a housedress with mismatched seams, who is wearing earrings I wouldn't wear and whose sweat smells old. Should I move? Would it be rude to move? (She smells of hard work, lazy old Cancer Bitch.)

I'm equally judgmental about women who wear stiletto heels, because they show bad sense, retro politics and misplaced vanity. Unless they are reading books that I think show evidence of a live intellect. A therapist once suggested that I look at people as works of art. I have taken figure drawing and I should be able to do this. But I am critical. Of just about everything. Most of the thought that is underneath my thought has to do with comparing. I am trying to figure out if this person (in paisley, for instance) is as fat as I am or fatter. This is what girls are trained to do. Our comparing comes

partly from our never being able to know exactly what we look like from the outside. Another part has to do with the patriarchy. The other other part has to do with keeping ourselves to ourselves. Yes, we are made of sand and ash like everybody else, but what if we really believed deep down to the bottom of our DNA that we were just made up of molecules and atoms and subatomic particles, just as everything and everyone else is—like this keyboard and the sidewalk and the person in paisley—would we then lose our outline? Would we merge with the rest of the world? Would our skin fly off and all our thoughts breeze away into the clouds?
 Perhaps.
 And that is why I am afraid of meditation.

September 14. Sins

    I threw my sins into the lake yesterday. It's a Rosh Hashanah custom. Usually we throw bread crumbs as a stand-in, but there's talk now that the crumbs could upset the ecosystem. So I threw a very few crumbs and some sand and some rocks. Seagulls found us and hovered and dove and one of them went after a rock I threw. I was glad the bird came up empty. It would be terrible to be responsible for killing a seagull while you were throwing off last year's sins. The synagogue I went to is unaffiliated, meaning it's not Reform or Conservative or Orthodox or Traditional or Conservadox or Reconstructionist or Renewal. Though it seems like Renewal. Stuff about breathing and light in the photocopied prayer book, and God isn't called He unless there's a reference to She coming up soon. I've never understood what's so revolutionary about making God genderless or hermaphroditic. To me the issue is God in general. I don't believe in God, though I've mellowed over the last year or so (not related to cancer) and can accept God as a label for the ineffable liveliness of the atoms inside each of us and everything around us. I was telling Linc about this last night and he said then who are you praying to? I said it's general gratitude. He said why do you need that? I said it makes you more grateful for what you have. He accepted that.

September 15. Here Comes the Fuzz

The thing is, we confuse recovery from chemo with recovery from cancer. So as my hair slowly grows back, I start to feel that I'm cured, that spring is in the air (though it's an autumnlike day, time to bring the basil crop inside). My scalp now feels like a tennis ball, according to Garnett, or peach fuzz, according to Linc. I have some dark stubs, too, on my scalp, along with a few wayward one-inch white hairs, and dark little dots on my otherwise pale eyebrow area, and my eyelashes are moving from sparse to less so.

My black head-decoration is wearing off in back. I will need a touch-up soon, though Linc says soon the fuzz on my head will keep the ink or henna from sticking. As if he knows. Even though I'm optimistic about the near-future return of my hair, I just sent off for more jagua ink, this time from a place in the UK instead of California, because of the lower price and the different shape of the container—a tube instead of a difficult-to-squeeze needle-nosed bottle.

September 16. Sadness, the Empty Room

We (I) spend time talking to Barry and Sharon, telling them what they should do, in light of Barry's MS getting worse, in light of his falls from his chair, and my nattering and nagging fill the air, fill the space, takes the place of emotion. But when Sharon talked about it last night, about Barry needing full-time help, or when I think about him in assisted living, I get overwhelmed by sadness. Yesterday he had a bad day, he could barely get out of bed. They realize how bad the situation is, and it changes the conversation. They finally see it as tragic and impossible as I do.

September 17. Homage to Our Podiatrist

Our podiatrist is avuncular. He is nice-looking with short white hair that sticks up. He has a Hungarian vizsla dog who is ageing (who does not come to the office). His staff unties your shoes and takes off your socks, and when the appointment is over, puts your socks on and ties up your shoes for you. The staff is like Mom and he is the avunc. His brother is in practice with him as well as a doctor who wears a yarmulke. Today there was a nun in the waiting room. Usually there is a rabbi. Our podiatrist will clip our nails. He seems happy to see me. He uses ultrasound and prolotherapy and has a fancy way of making orthotics involving gait, he doesn't just put your feet into a sticky substance to make the mold. He gives me samples of Biofreeze to massage into my Achilles tendon. He believes in vitamin B for circulation. In the waiting room is a plaque acknowledging his father's efforts in getting podiatry accepted as a bonafide part of the medical profession, complete with insurance reimbursement. The father and the two sons practiced together. Now it is just the two sons. Our podiatrist has two sons and one is in screenwriting and the other is in Israel. That son is fluent in Hebrew. Our podiatrist has that Jewish-Skokie accent that sounds almost like New York-Yiddish-inflected. He is comforting in his goodlookingness and uncle/fatherliness and his confidence. Most of all his confidence. He tries this then he tries that. He is calm about trying this then that, scientific method, tick this off, then that. Our podiatrist's synagogue is fifty years old and has had the same rabbi that whole time. On Rosh Hashanah our podiatrist threw his sins into the canal. Our podiatrist stands for stability and family and father-sonliness and Skokie, though he practices in Chicago. He seems to come out of an earlier time, when sons followed into their fathers' businesses, when it wasn't so hard to find people. By that I mean, people didn't stray so far from their origins. I do mean it was easier to locate people. They stayed where they belonged. I didn't stay where I belonged. But the podiatrist makes me feel that I have come into a place where everyone has remained for a generation a two, where they are settled but will move over for a newcomer or two. Where there is a place. Where there will always be a place.

September 21. Bikram Kol Nidre

O man, was it hot in services tonight. We had an *erev* (eve) Yom Kippur dinner here and then three of us went to the little congregation that meets in a church. There were two ceiling fans and one rotating fan. I wanted to go stand by the rotating fan but didn't want to hog the air. I have been a very sweaty Cancer Bitch it seems like forever. Partly it's because I stopped taking black cohosh because it interferes with one of my Pills to Combat Melancholy. Partly it's from being zapped from peri-menopause into full-blown menopause by the chemo. Partly, according to my acupuncturist, it's because I'm still getting rid of the toxins. When I get warm, I stay very very warm. And get sweaty. When I have a slightly unpleasant thought or think of a time when I was embarrassed or irritated, I get sweaty. I get a clammy fuzzy head and then sweat streams and streams around my face. And then too when I'm just sitting around or standing or walking, calm and minding my own business, a flash starts. Sometimes I feel my ears get red first. I don't mind the heat, it's the sweat. I can't take soy for the flashes because of the cancer. The cancer (the cancer that is no longer with us, the cancer that was cut out with wide margins, the cancer that was sliced and diced and put in paraffin) feeds on estrogen and estrogen-like substances, such as pesticides and possibly soy, and possibly recombinant bovine growth hormone. Which means I eat organic as much as possible, soy as little as possible. (Though experts are divided about the soy.)

But back to the holiest day of the year. Erev Yom Kippur services are called Kol Nidre after the first prayer which is chanted three times. My father always said, Kol Nidre can make or break a cantor. I thought that was funny. Our family tradition was to wisecrack during services. Tonight we got to services late, after the Kol Nidre. I think the real reason it is repeated is so that latecomers will get to hear it. Forgive me, I missed the Kol Nidre at the Kol Nidre service.

We confess on behalf of the community: We have done this, we have done that. But our prayers, repentance and charity will help us be forgiven. Every year we say we are sorry. And then we go out and sin some more. We are supposed to ask forgiveness of people we have sinned against. But I am stubborn. I am unchanging. I had a best friend, Amelia. I don't have her any more. I should ask forgiveness for hurting her. Did I hurt her? I still feel competitive with her. Is that a sin? Yes. A sin against her, against me, against the universe. If I am competitive, it means there is not enough. It means that I am paying too much attention to what she has. I am looking to the side when I should look ahead. Or inside. I do rejoice when other friends rejoice. I am not always ungenerous. I should ask forgiveness for the times I provoked her. For being late. For staying annoyed. For holding a grudge. We have held grudges, we have bribed, we have betrayed, we have cheated, we have stolen. Forgive us, all of us. We are sorry. By tradition, we beat our chests while we confess, but the modern adaptation is to massage our hearts—after all, we are of the generation that believes in not beating yourself up. Just as we no longer give one another thirty-nine (light, according to tradition) lashes. Massage your heart until it produces regret. Massage your heart until it is soft, and warmth radiates from it, settling on all the bits and pieces and the big large things in the universe. Massage your heart until it opens. It is a hard heart. It is a frightened heart. It is afraid that if it opens like a locket and takes in the universe, it will disappear. It is afraid that it will then become the universe's heart. It will no longer be the heart of the one, the only Cancer Bitch. It will be just like anybody else's. But it already looks like anybody else's. It pumps blood. It does all the things a heart does. Its blood is type O+, which is the most common type, the type that billions of other humans have and had and will have. Its blood can be given, though not universally. Its blood can be sorted and separated and centrifuged and spread between clear glass plates. It can be spilled. (*If you prick us, do we not bleed?*)

One story about Eden, said the rabbi, is that Adam and Eve were pure light. And then when they were exiled from the garden they were given skins. To contain them, to separate them from every other thing in the world that they had not been separate from. Another story is that everything in the world was made of light. Then the light became fragmented and we are trying in this life to collect and connect all the light, to restore and repair the world.

The way to heal, I think, and I mean heal the soul, is to train yourself to see the light everywhere. Until you know without looking. Until you feel it without pointing it out to yourself, mouthing the words. It's just there. Like it's been all along.

◆ ◆ ◆

A few hours after I wrote this I realized: I wanted too much from Amelia. I wanted too much and didn't tell her and then the resentment started. And when I told her, the resentment had already taken root. For all that I am sorry.

September 22. The Right Side

The weather was cool today, so it was Yom Kippur without that Bikram feeling. I had scheduled my arrival to services just about right: I got to the little-synagogue-that-isn't-there at about 1:30 pm, with just two prayers to go before the break.

At the break I talked to a man who told me his wife had died of breast cancer. It bothers me to look at you, he said, because of it. She was fifty when she was diagnosed, and had ten years before it came back. How old are you, he said, in your twenties? I'm fifty-one, I said. When I told him the cancer was not in my lymph nodes, he gestured dismissively, as if I had nothing to worry about. I also talked with an androgynous eighteen-year-old diabetic who was fasting, but who had brought insulin and food just in case. I said I was fasting but I was drinking water. Did your oncologist tell you to do that? the young person asked. No, I said, my husband did. The diabetic said, When I was diagnosed, the first thing I wanted to know was if I could fast on Yom Kippur.

September 23. Four Women, Four Breasts

I went to Ann and Peggy's 30th anniversary picnic today. When they were cutting the cake I was standing nearby, and noticed Nancy (mastectomy) standing on Ann's other side. Later I said to Ann (mastectomy): I don't think I've been anywhere where there were three one-breasted women. And then she pointed out a fourth. Ann, Nancy and I don't wear prostheses. Ann, Nancy and the fourth woman are all lesbians. Are lesbians less likely to opt for reconstruction? Are they less attached to the symmetry that epitomizes the mainstream male-centered female ideal? Earlier, I was waiting on the corner for Garnett to give me a ride to the picnic. The Cubs game was just letting out.

A guy noticed my adorned baldness and exclaimed: Look at you!

What would he have said if he'd noticed my one-breastedness? Depends on how drunk he was.

September 25. What is Mine

Marcel Marceau is mine. And that's not a typo. He is mine because his father, Karl Mangel, was born in a small town in Poland and was a kosher butcher in Strasbourg. I understand kosher butchers. I understand Yiddish-speaking Polish fathers, though mine wasn't either. After his father was arrested, Marcel and his brother worked in the Resistance. Marcel took a new last name from a Victor Hugo poem. He used his artistic skill to forge documents. He led a group of Jewish children, dressed as Boy Scouts, across the Swiss frontier. He took drama lessons in Paris from a school that had been named, before and after the War, for a famous Jewish actress. Sarah Bernhardt (who also identified as Catholic). She is mine, too. So is Simone Weil; and Edith Piaf, but only because I saw the Piaf movie. Simone de Beauvoir isn't mine, though I know she had an orgasm for the first time when she had sex with Nelson Algren on the beach in Indiana. He isn't mine, either, though he was Jewish. Or maybe it was in his apartment in Chicago. She wrote him love letters.

Marceau's father was murdered in Auschwitz, and so was Karl's younger brother.

Herschel Grynzspan is mine. Anne Frank is mine, though she's everyone's and they've all trooped through her cramped re-created attic in Amsterdam. Philip Roth is mine, though Cynthia Ozick is not. I.B. Singer is not, Bernard Malamud is not, though he was my teacher's teacher, and my teacher named his son after him. Delmore Schwartz is mine. St. Augustine is mine, for his agony, though I haven't read his diary since freshman year of college. So is Thomas Merton. Both had wild early years. Charlotte Salomon is mine, and Lincoln Park (the neighborhood) is mine. Louis Sullivan is mine—the ornamentation, not the shape of the buildings—and Sacagawea and Edna St. Vincent Millay, whose former summer place I stayed in for a month on a fellowship. Squirrels are mine, and raccoons, and dachshunds and beagles. Cicada skins and doodle bugs and grasshoppers, though they struggle against my closed hand (quick as lightning) and spit tobacco juice on my fingers. Lightning bugs aren't mine. Mark Twain isn't mine though he looks so familiar in his white mustache and suit. Milk chocolate is mine, but only when it's sold in bulk, and covers almonds or malt balls. Milk shakes aren't mine though chocolate chip ice cream is. Tiropita is mine. And kosher gumbo. And espresso. Organic milk is mine, and organic rice milk. Dark wood molding is mine, and green walls against dark wood is mine, and also polished light pine floors. Dark chocolate is never mine. French is mine and Hebrew is mine, and spoken but not written Yiddish. Kafka is mine. The Nora Ephron from the seventies is mine. Mrs. Pigglewiggle is and so is Jeanne-Marie who counts her sheep. Little Brown Bear is mine and Judy Bolton but not Nancy Drew.

Emma Goldman is mine and Eugene Debs and the Abraham Lincoln Brigade. Frida Kahlo and Walter Benjamin are mine but I have to share them with everybody else. New York isn't mine but Berkeley is. And Venice, though I don't know it well, and twisty little rue Mouffetard, with its Vietnamese and Moroccan restaurants in the late 1970s, is mine. *Adon Olam* is mine and *Avenu Malkenu*. The year 1968 isn't mine, or 1967, but 1945 is and 1976 and 1978. Crosswords aren't mine, nor Scrabble nor Monopoly, but Clue is. Barcelona isn't mine though I walked its streets and into its Art Nouveau lobbies for almost a week. Harbors aren't mine. Nor boats. Cambridge, Mass., is mine. And Newport, R.I. Lapis lazuli is mine but not jade or silver. Nail polish isn't mine but bow lips are. Silent films aren't mine but Tina Modotti is. *Der Blaue Engel* is mine though I don't understand German. Potato latkes are mine though I don't fry things well. Mary McCarthy is mine. The Bayeux Tapestry is almost mine. Glowworms are almost mine. The main square in Brussels is mine, though I've been there just once. South Street in Philadelphia is mine. Whole Foods and Trader Joe's aren't mine, though I seem to be in one or the other every other day. The sun is not mine but the two-thirds-full moon is. Pansies are, especially dark ones.

Why must I claim so much? Why must I own, even in words?

I saw Marcel Marceau, wide-eyed and white-faced, perform in Chicago. I couldn't see what he was seeing. Maybe, he said to an interviewer, I am silent because of the silence of those who returned from the camps. But this was not his own idea; he was saying Perhaps in answer to the journalist's question.

The amoeba makes itself an arm so it can reach what it wants. The amoeba surrounds the thing and takes it into its one-celled self.

Everything is already named. I have been alive for half a century. I do not know what to do with myself.

September 29. Hairline

I look like Sluggo, Nancy's pal in the comic strip. My hairline is lower than my tattoo-line was, and I look like a Neanderthal. My tattoos are mostly faded. I want to get someone to rewrite the US out of Iraq on the back of my head. My scalp still shows through the hair. My eyebrows are growing in but I still use pencil to darken them. My eyes are close together (an oculist told me, and it's true) and I think it's more pronounced now that the tattoos are gone. I am vain and obsessed. I think about 50 percent of the time about my hair/non-hair and the rest of the time about food, students, writing, the world brutality *du jour*, cancer coming back. Not in that order. The order keeps changing. I applied today for a fellowship from the Isherwood Foundation. I didn't mention my breast cancer on the personal statement. What could I say? I have breast cancer, feel sorry for me and send money, my time may be short? But think of all the writers with AIDS who may be applying. Breast cancer seems like chump change in comparison. At least my kind of. Maybe that is why my oncologist (soon to be my former) seemed bored with it. Or maybe he is without affect. I will see the new young female oncologist on Friday. The old oncologist seemed indifferent to my case. He didn't call my Bouncy Shrink back to talk about drug interactions and when they did talk (after she called again) she asked him about monitoring my liver something or other and he brushed her off. I want an oncologist who at least feigns interest.

September 30. Genes and Hormones

I found out Thursday I don't have the BRCA gene mutations, more common in Ashkenazi Jews than the general population. That mutation predisposes the bearer to breast and ovarian cancer. I didn't think I had it, but wanted to make sure, and the genetic counselor had said I had an 18 percent chance of having it. She's still waiting to see if I have a certain other mutation responsible for breast and uterine cancer. I need to get her one more piece of information before she can tell me that I'm a suspect. And if I am? I guess a hysterectomy will follow. Does this never end?

Recently I was talking to a student about academic matters, and then she said, You're my age, aren't you? and I am, and she turned the talk to menopause and hot flashes. Hers sound worse, only because she doesn't have a partner, so that she's been on dates when she's broken out in a sweat. At least I don't have to be embarrassed about them when I'm with Linc. How many times have I asked him, Is it hot in here? And we know the answer: No, it's just me. I'm like a kid who keeps saying: You know what? That's what!

October 1. Cancer Bitch Turns a Corner & Runs Into a Wall

Tonight I looked in the mirror and thought to myself, You are cute. I think I have just passed the awkward Sluggo stage and am now a boyish woman in a shorter-than-crew cut. I even have most of my eyebrows back. I am surprised that in all this time, no one's thought I was male. I did have girly-feminine designs atop my scalp and I usually wear two earrings, not the lone little hoop that often signifies Cool Male Who Dares to Pierce One Ear. But approached from the left, I am flat-chested. Then again, I do have a female voice. Last month the young person I met at synagogue asked me if anyone thought I was gay because of my short/non-existent hair. I told this young person that only at the Whole Foods I might have been eyed a few times by women, but that's probably because it's attached to a new LGBT community center.

When I was talking to this young person I was dying to know this person's gender— I, who was all prepared to have people ask me whether I was male or female, and to respond tartly: Why does it matter? Yes, I wanted to know whether this short, slight person— with about 1/8-inch-long hair under a cap, body swallowed by a baggy long-sleeved white shirt tucked into loose pants—was male or female. Why? Why is it so disconcerting not to know? Why couldn't I just have a conversation with a Person? Years ago, my friend Robin and his then-wife returned from his seven-month fellowship in Provincetown. I remember the erstwhile wife saying she'd been taken aback by all the gay men in P-town. This is what she said bothered her: She was used to speaking to men in a certain way (flirtily, I guess?), and being noticed by men in a certain way, and these men (in stores, for example) were responding differently (or maybe she said not responding). This surprised me. I figured I didn't expect as much as she did from men in casual encounters. But I'm not very flirty. Sometimes, though, I feel my eyes widen when I'm speaking to a man who's in possession of stereotypically male expertise—mostly having to do with appliances and automobiles. I guess I sink into the O, what do I know? housewifey mode. I am stereotypically female when it comes to home repairs and hardware, and I'm not proud of this ignorance. But I come by it honestly. My mother didn't change ceiling light bulbs, and as for my father— changing light bulbs was the extent of household expertise. That and killing cockroaches. Linc changes the difficult high light bulbs because when I use the extender thing I break the bulbs. I kill silverfish and roaches myself. I let spiders out. The other day at the dentist's I noticed a spider, and he caught it in a cup and I let it out on a planter on Michigan Avenue.

But I am moving away from the uncomfortable subject of the young person of uncertain gender.

Later in conversation I found out that the person was transgender, born a girl, identifying as male. And only eighteen. OK, that explained everything, I was no longer uneasy. I solved the mystery. But there's still the mystery of why I was uneasy in the first place, why I needed the answer to the question: What are you?

I know that we classify people, and that we routinely ask the gender of the baby in the passing stroller, and even the dog walking by on the leash. And I know that I want to ask, Where are you from? each time I hear an accent. But why? Because we have certain ideas about what constitutes male and female, and male and female characteristics, and what it means if the person speaking to us is from Poland or Germany (*Ossi* or *Wessi*?) and I know I bring certain assumptions if I know my interlocutor is Jewish.

I won't answer this now because I can't. I will only say that in the summer of 1992 I was in Krakow, Poland, and I was looking for the building where a Jewish girls' boarding school had been housed before the War. It was now a school for the deaf. There was a caretaker couple that was not hearing-impaired, but they didn't speak English and I don't speak Polish. We made do in pidgin German, and using gestures and drawings. I managed to understand that the granddaughter of a former student had visited, and that the couple was going to let me in and look around. School was out for the summer. They asked me, *Was sind Sie*? What are you? American, I answered disingenuously. I knew that wasn't what they were asking. But I wouldn't tell them I was Jewish. Why? Because I didn't want them to know. Or to know for certain. Why? Was it because I didn't want them to think that only Jews were interested in the history of the building, and thus, the history of Jews? Maybe.

October 7. The Curly-Haired Oncologist

Linc went with me to the appointment with the new oncologist. Two hours after the time of the initial appointment, she came in. She made the mistake of asking how I was. I told her. I said I was annoyed at having to wait so long. She said she was sorry and that she'd spent fifteen to twenty minutes looking up possible drug interactions on my behalf. She touched me on the leg when she walked in and while she was talking to me. It seemed a little scripted. (Touch patient to establish humanity.)

After she left, Linc said I shouldn't switch again. You've already burned one bridge (oncologist #1), he said. I don't want to keep having appointments with new oncologists. He went back to work and called a couple of hours later. He asked how I was. Angry, I said. You can be a little angry, he said, but you shouldn't be very angry. I can be however angry I want, I said.

October 9. Hyper

Days like this I think I'm manic. I've been sleeping a lot probably still because of chemo, and I keep sleeping later and later and then I have to get up early some time and I screw up my inner clock. Last night I went to bed late but this morning I couldn't sleep. I got up early (meaning, in the single digits). I met with a private writing student and had an iced latte with rice milk. I wrote e-mails. I'm feeling that I'm writing too many e-mails. Do the receivers discern my franticness? Do they think I'm irrational, beyond caffeinated? When I don't get enough sleep I am hyper. I get drunk on not-enough sleep. I lived like this for most of high school. Diet Dr. Peppers, NoDoz, five hours of sleep a night on weeknights and a visit to the ophthalmologist: Why do I have headaches? I asked.

There was always a lump in my throat because—well, partly because I was nervous and irritable from not enough sleep—and partly because that is my nature. As I've said before, I take several pills now keep to melancholia and despair at bay. Those pills were just a glimmer in an R&D researcher's eye back when I was in high school. On weekends I would sleep twelve, fourteen hours. Weeknights I stayed at school until 2 a.m. working on the semiweekly school paper. We worked in a separate little building (one of the *shacks*) on campus, which had a Selectric typewriter, printing machine, couch, fridge, and a closet in which a stray cat had given birth. The editors had keys and I was an editor. The main school building closed at 10:00 pm or so. Once around 1:00 am we went inside the building to use the bathroom and set off the alarm. The cops came. Several cars of them. Probably all of the police cars that existed in the little suburb where the school was. I lived in the city of Houston, but the school was in Bellaire, which was surrounded by the city.

We had to call the principal on the pay phone to vouch for us. And he did. He knew us. Then we went home. We were outraged but amused. When the other editor and I went away to (the same) college, the principal gave us $20 so we could go out for a nice meal. That was back when $20 could get you a fancy meal for two. Or maybe it was $10. It was a long time ago.

In high school I was miserable because of the anxious lump in my throat, and because I wasn't accepted into an Ivy League school (Both Linc and I were wait-listed at Brown, in different years. We're both still waiting for our numbers to come up.), but underneath the anxiety I had a good time, if that makes sense. And my friends and I were very lucky; I drank beer with some girls during lunch one day and we came back and played a very giggly and spirited volleyball game in gym class and we weren't caught. On Saturday nights we had parties at the houses of friends whose parents were out of town and we didn't get caught. We didn't know you shouldn't drink and drive, the admonition hadn't been invented yet. At a party a friend passed out and finally at 5:00 am or so the rest of us decided we had to get him up and out. Somehow we maneuvered him into his car and we followed him as he slowly, very slowly, drove home. How could we? But he made it home. A few years later he realized he was an alcoholic and quit drinking. But not in high school. Excess wasn't recognized as such then. Except there was a boy who was going to be a doctor and he got very drunk and rammed his car and became paralyzed. We don't know what happened to him next. At all.

October 15. Good News, Sort Of

US cancer rates are on the decline, a group of scientists announced today. In further good news, the AP reports: *New breast cancer diagnoses are dropping about 3.5 percent a year....* It's either because fewer post-menopausal women are opting for hormone replacement therapy, or—here's the punch line—fewer women are getting mammograms.

Maybe that's one reason that there is more breast cancer in developed countries than developing: because women in the former are less likely to have access to the machines that detect early cancers. Another reason might be that those women aren't exposed to as many carcinogens as in industrialized nations (though I know the air is bad in some developing countries.). Or they die of other causes.

If we ever get national health insurance, and the rates soar, we'll know it was the access problem.

October 16. Hair-Dos and Don'ts

Tonight I received a teaching award from Smart U. First there was a reception, during which I had my second Very Hot Flash of the Day while standing near some hot hors d'oeuvres. Luckily I was had on Hot Flash Defensivewear (silk scarf tied around my hairline) to catch some of the sweat. As I was standing around I saw a woman come into the room with my exact hairdo. I assumed she was a sister chemo-head and I felt immediate affinity. Even her salt-to-pepper ratio was very much like mine. I went up to her and said, I had to talk to you because your hair's like mine. She said, Is your haircut intentional? And I said no. I asked her and she said yes. I felt immediately stupid. I felt that I had insulted her: No one would have hair like ours unless she couldn't help it. I didn't get a chance to finish talking to her, to say, It looks good on you, I don't think it looks good on me.

Students nominate faculty for the award, and then the deans look up your teaching evaluations and discuss you and decide who gets honored. I was pleased to get the award, even as I suspected it was a sympathy vote. I have been teaching college for twenty-one years and still I get insecure. And of course I still make mistakes. After the ceremony I went to teach a class at Brain Trust University and we went off on a tangent and I was leading the way. In a distinguished manner, of course.

October 21. All Her Life

My mother came in last weekend to Cancer Bitch World HQ. My mother would have flown in for every chemo treatment, but I wouldn't let her. I asked if she would help me with my clutter, and she agreed. So we spent most of Saturday and Sunday going through photos. We filled some albums and threw a lot of pictures away. We pasted some pictures in my baby book, which she'd apparently lost interest in after my first full sentence. She's been diligent about collecting pictures in albums, though—I don't mean to imply that she ever lost interest in recording moments of my life. My mother didn't fill this book, I think, because she put photos of my first birthday party in an album, followed by other family photos. Most of us don't think to take one photo from each event or year or decade and paste it into a baby or any other kind of book.

But what if we did? What if every New Year's Eve we printed out a couple of representative photos from our desktops and put them in a book, a book with a finite number of bound pages? Is that too frightening to contemplate? My baby book is called *All Her Life*. When you get to the end, you're ded. Or sitting in the nursing home, with no one thinking to take your picture or record your first dentures, your first wheelchair, your last meal cooked for yourself, your last wisp of short-term memory.

November 26. Losing Days and Years

Once I asked an E.B. White scholar why White's essay, "Once More to the Lake," is so much anthologized and taught, and he answered: Because it's the best essay in the English language. Or something to that effect. Which may be why I'm calling it to mind. I guess a great piece of writing is one that you call to mind to encapsulate your own experiences, among other things. White writes about going to the lake in the summer as a boy and going back as a father, and that slippage that happens in which everything about the place seems eternal, and he doesn't know any more if he's the boy or the father or what year it is. That same feeling is in Thornton Wilder's play *The Long Christmas Dinner*. It all takes place at, well, a Christmas dinner table, and it's populated by generations of a family. The members grow old and die (walk offstage) and younger family members (who look more or less like their forebears) come to the table and grow older. Some repeat the phrases of the elders. When we come together for a holiday, the same place, the same people (more or less), it's like one long event, punctuated by your life outside.

Last week I stayed at the preposterously spelled Hilton Lincoln Centre in Dallas, which used to be the DoubleTree, just as I have for I don't know how long. At the gargantuan Thanksgiving buffet there was the same ice sculpture of a turkey and the same thawed shrimp and crab claws as in years past, and I remembered my great-aunt Ethel heaping her plate with shrimp, and others remembered our cousin Chad piling everything on his plate, back before he became glatt kosher and stopped eating anything in non-kosher places. Aunt Ethel died several years ago, and, eerily, after she died, I received a Jewish new year's card from her. There was a note inside from her daughter, explaining that she'd found it on her mother's desk.

December 1. *In Medias Res*

This is the third year in a row that the grad students in my teaching seminar are holding a weekend of free creative writing classes for the public. I came up with the idea my very own Cancer Bitch self and it is a very nice thing for everyone involved. No one pays a thing. The students get the experience of creating and teaching 50-minute classes to strangers, and the strangers get the free classes. This year someone on staff did the messy work of taking registrations and putting the class lists on a spreadsheet, making much less work for me.

I like very much being in the middle of everything. In the middle of the hallway of the university-owned mansion where the classes are held, sitting at a table and listening to the class going on while I grade papers. The floor is hardwood and there's molding on the walls and fancy lighting fixtures hanging down and one room that's a 19th-century parlor in greens and reds. I like being in the mansion, and being the person in charge. During the week when I happen to go to the building, it's filled with people doing their jobs and there is no desk for Cancer Bitch. There is no place at school for me to display my etched crystal teaching award. I used to have a cubicle on the top floor but I hardly ever used it so it was snatched away from me. So that is my own fault. I do have a cabinet in the back of the cubicle. And a mail box, which has disappeared only once.

In the mansion this time of year there's a little light-up Christmas village on a window sill. A friend who works there thinks it should be an authentic Dickensian city, complete with prostitutes, pickpockets and paupers. As soon as someone can figure out how to market that version, I'm sure we'll see it in stores.

December 2. Teaching One-Breasted

Today was the second and last day of the writing workshops led by my students. I had to fill in for one of them for about thirty minutes today. I was wearing a long-sleeved hot pink shirt that clearly hugs my right breast and left non-breast. I'd been wearing it all day but hadn't spent much time in front of a crowd, though I had made quick announcements all day. I felt like there was something obscene about revealing my lack of breast in public. Which is interesting. Nipples have been considered obscene, and that accounts for the tassels worn by go-go dancers. Pubic hair has been considered obscene, and thus the merkin was invented, a small wig that exotic dancers could use to cover their pubic hair. Which is absurd. I don't know why pubic hair is obscene in the first place, because it's the stuff that *covers* the genitals.

I felt like I was flaunting my one-breastedness, while at the same time I felt defiant: Hey, world, this is what breast cancer looks like. If one in seven or eight women will have breast cancer at some point in their lives, and if some of these women (I don't know what percent) will have a breast cut out, slashed and scooped, amputated, what have you—then it seems that one-breasted women would therefore be fixtures in our grocery stores, offices, restaurants, classrooms and so on. Of course, they are all around us but they're wearing prostheses. Or they've had reconstruction and have been restored to double-breastedness. I don't know what percent opts for reconstruction. I don't even know if I'm going to opt for reconstruction. It seems by now that I've always had only one breast.

And I don't know the stats for women who've had double mastectomies.

You might say that the women who have replaced their breasts permanently or temporarily are opting for privacy. Or you could say they're being dishonest by covering up the results of surgery. You could also say that their breasts are a lot bigger than mine, and you'd be right. How defiant would I be if I had a flatness on one side, and on the other side had a breast the size of a child's head?

December 3. Library Cancer Card

I'm in the midst of checking out a book at the Smart U library, and the clerk tells me my account is blocked because I owe $200. Which can't be. Because faculty don't get fines. So then the finance person comes out and I tell her I renewed everything on line, and she says you can renew books just twice now, not forever and ever, and now faculty are being fined, and that my Juno e-mail account wasn't accepting the overdue notices from the library. I decide it's time to use the cancer card, especially since she's wearing a pink ribbon pin. She says I look familiar and I say I remember talking to her about the Holocaust, and I say I used to look different, I had more hair, before I had a chemo cut. And she says, How are you? And I say fine, not even feeling guilty for my calculated cancer insert. Because what is cancer good for if not to help a person get out of paying fines?

And it works. She gives me a break, letting me check out a book and telling me I need to return three books to the library (Help me help you, she says), which I'll do on Thursday when I go to class.

At home two other books have been sitting on the dining room table for a long long time and they belong to the public library of Chicago. This is why I buy books. I had my Brain Trust U students read that Grace Paley story, Wants, about a woman who is returning books to the library that are eighteen years overdue, and she writes a check to cover her $32 in fines. Paley writes: *Immediately* [the librarian] *trusted me, put my past behind her, wiped the record clean, which is just what most other municipal and/or state bureaucracies will not do.*

December 9. The Fear

The fear, the fear always of not amounting to anything. That's one way of saying it. I fear I will not, I do not, amount to anything. Meaning I am nothing?

We are all nothing. We are all here for a moment.

Fame. Ambition. Strive to create work as excellent at Dante's, as poet Donald Hall says. Not to be famous. Not to become known. But to create work that is sui generis. It is the work, not the life that is important. Though we confuse the art with the life, and fall in love with pitiful (we think) Kafka because of his life.

Wasting time fits in here somewhere. The restlessness of time-wasting. The nothingness of it. The nothing-to-show-for-it-ness of it. Wasting time means that you are not making something. You are making nothing. Spinning your wheels. The wheels are not attached to anything. They're not making anything go. They're not turning straw into gold.

December 19. The Phancy Phlebotomist

I had a blood test today on Ye Olde Cancer Floor at Fancy Hospital. The phlebotomists have always been nice and personable and usually talkative. The phlebotomist I was assigned to was setting things up today when another phlebotomist came by eating a shortbread cookie. The two of them talked about how tempting they were, and then my phlebotomist said she doesn't mean to eat cookies and such but as soon as she sees them, she eats them. We commiserated about all the tempting foods out and about at this time of year and she told me she had to stop eating so much because she didn't want her New Year's Eve dress to be so tight on her that she looked like a whore, pardon my French. She told me she'd bought a dress on sale Marshall Field's in October or November five years ago, for $85, and it had sequins and ruffles on top and two tiers of material below her knees. It was going to be her New Year's Eve dress. But when the time came to put it on, it was too tight: Girl, she said, it looked like I had four titties and six booties.

January 1. The New Year

We went to Barry and Sharon's for New Year's Eve, as we've done for many years, and as I did for years before meeting Linc. The guests vary a little from year to year, but there are stalwarts. Sometimes it is a sit-down dinner and sometimes it's not. Once it was a barbecue and they turned the heat up and wore Hawaiian shirts. Now we are all battered. Barry was in his wheelchair, of course, and I looked around and thought: Last year I had cancer but didn't know it. Among the people here are two pairs of parents whose sons have died, and I wonder what suffering is in store for all of us; in what new ways will we be damaged by the time we're together for the next New Year's Eve? I thought, this is like Walter Benjamin's image of the angel of history, who looks into the past and sees only one large tragedy unfolding, except in this case I'm looking forward and seeing a road tragedy up ahead.

January 4. Causes, not Cures

Jack the environmental activist sent this to me:

> No matter how much our efforts to treat cancer may advance, the best way to reduce cancer's toll is to keep people from getting it. We need to join the rest of the industrialized world by issuing a national ban on asbestos and forbidding smoking in the workplace and other public spaces. We must reduce the hazards faced by those working to build our homes, transport our goods and make the products we consume. We should restrict CT scans of children to medical emergencies, limit the use of diagnostic radiation in general, ban young children from using cellphones and keep the rest of us from using tanning beds. And we must recognize that pollutants do not need passports. Controlling cancer, like controlling global warming, can take place only on an international scale.
> —*University of Pittsburgh's Graduate School of Public Health, November 4, 2007, quoted on cancerprevention society.org*

January 15. Worry and Not Worry

I fell on my back about a month ago in step aerobics. This may seem impossible, but I did. We were sitting on our risers or whatever you call those long flat boards, holding those colored stretchy bands with handles. My legs were straight and the band was around my feet, but then slipped off and I fell back. I wasn't hurt much. This is only important because I still have some pain (mostly when I push at the sites) around one vertebra and on my coccyx. And the pain wouldn't be important except that when cancer metastasizes it goes to the bones and shows itself as pain. I'm worried/not worried about it. I had a check-up appointment today with the surgeon. Her physician's assistant pushed on the places, hard, and said that if it was cancer, most likely it would have hurt more than it did. They both said that if the pain doesn't go away in a month, to call and get an X-ray. Deep down, I think it's nothing.

People ask me if there are scans to see if the cancer has come back, and there are, but the booklet the oncologist gave me (and which I can't find at the moment) says that there's no reason to do scans all the time, that mostly women report pain or other symptoms that turn out to be cancer. If I had the pain and I hadn't fallen in aerobics, I would be really worried. It does seem rather fast for metastasis. Chemo ended only five months ago, and the chances of cancer coming back *without chemo* was only 30 percent. How dare it come back so quickly?

January 16. Anniversary: The Ritual Crushing of the Pills

On January 16 a year ago, the radiologist at the Mammogram Factory was pretty grim as she looked at my ultrasound and told me I needed an ultrasound-guided core-needle biopsy. And so the fun began.

I decided that the best way to commemorate this event was to grind up the pills that I'd been issued for chemo side-effects. I mean, my understanding is that I can't have any more chemo, and if there were some kind of chemo for me in the future, I'm sure the doctors would issue newerbetterstrongerlongerlasting pills to take.

The party couldn't start till 10:00 because I had class tonight. It's hard to get people to come to a party on a Wednesday night that begins at 10:00, especially when first advertised as providing no refreshments and lasting only fifteen minutes. I loosened up but the damage was done. Only our loyal *voisins de palier* came (We know where they live) and we drank champagne, ate cheese and crackers and vegetable dumplings, and crushed the pills. Linc bought me flowers. My neighbor Anand wanted me to put the resulting powder in an urn. Or burn it. Or sell it on the street. I gathered the bits into a pill bottle and put it in a gold mesh bag and I'm not sure what I'll do with it. I think it should stay enclosed so that it doesn't immediately contaminate the lake. My friend Don sent me a study not long ago about fish containing Prozac because people excreted the drugs, which went into the water supply. Really, what's the harm? Just a littler gentler fish and human population. And what's wrong with that?

January 20. Replacing, Refilling, Ending, Not Ending

The New York Times reported on Thursday about problems with breast implants. First of all, they don't last and have to be replaced. Second of all, they can leak and spill and scar. All good reasons not to have an implant, Linc said, reading over my shoulder. But you notice women's breasts, I said. I didn't marry you for your breasts, he said. He's against all elective surgery. But wants me to do what I want to do.

I sound like I'm arguing in favor of implants. I kept thinking I would have an implant after I got down to my ideal weight, because if you get an implant and lose weight, the breast stays the same size. But the more and more I live with one breast, the more natural it seems. And the more I hear about how you always feel the implant floating inside you, the less inclined I am to get the surgery. And if you get reconstruction using your belly fat, it's safer but requires a long operation and recovery. And you have a big scar across your stomach. I do have the requisite raw material, though.

I have to admit that I've been feeling lazy for not replacing my breast. Maybe feeling lazy and slatternly for going around braless and one-breastless. O gosh, lost a breast and didn't even sew one back on. As if it were a button fallen off a coat.

January 24. One Mastectomy, To Go

You've no doubt heard of drive-by surgeries—the derisive term coined by health reformers for inadequate hospital stays mandated or permitted by health insurance companies. I thought of fast mastectomies as I read a profile of photographer Lee Miller (1907-1977) in the January 21 *New Yorker*. In Paris, she took jobs that her mentor and lover Man Ray passed down to her. One of these assignments was to take pictures of operations at the Sorbonne medical school. The year was 1930. We're told: *Having watched a mastectomy, she asked the surgeon if she could keep the amputated breast. She arrived for a fashion shoot at the studio of French* Vogue *in a buoyant mood, carrying this grisly trophy on a dinner plate, then photographed it at a place setting, next to a knife and fork.* Serve that at your next dinner party, Judy Chicago!

The two small contact prints of a breast on a white plate were shown for the first time in a recent retrospective at the Victoria and Albert Museum. The show ended earlier this month. Miller's son told the *Times* of London a different story: she was in the operating room not on assignment, but because she was having an affair with the surgeon. The doctor invited her to take pictures and gave her the breasts, plural, because she asked for them. (As a sign of his love? Did the patient on the operating table wonder where her breasts had gone, could she have imagined that what had been inside of her would suddenly be put on a plate like the head of John the Baptist? That woman is the unknown soldier.)

Opines the Times: For years [Miller] had been celebrated for the beauty of her breasts. At one time, her breasts had even inspired the design of a champagne glass. Images of her face and body, particularly her breasts, had been snipped up by Man Ray as part of his reductive process of control. 'What did all that do to her, I wonder,' says [son Tony] Penrose 'The knowledge that men loved her body. Here she was, saying, "OK, you revere breasts. OK, here's one. Have it. Eat it."

And the shoot took place in the Vogue studio, where the commodification of women occurred every day. How easy it is to offer someone else's breasts.

These days, a photographer couldn't run off with someone's breasts hot off the body. Can you imagine? Stop, thief! Once I was in a restaurant and the waitress told us someone had come into the kitchen and made off with half our pizza. But breasts?

How wrong it feels to have parts of ourselves that never see the light—to have them taken from inside of us and looked at.

We have bones and muscles to hold our organs in place, so they don't go flopping around inside us, and we have skin so that everything won't fall out of us. There is something horrible about seeing what should be enclosed and encased and hidden by skin.

In Israel there are Orthodox volunteers who gather body parts after a bombing to make sure that the remains have a religious burial. For them, every particle of a human is sacred.

What did that woman look like, the one who lay on the table at the Sorbonne medical school while another woman made sport of her breasts? Did that woman live? We assume her breasts were cancerous and were removed in order to save her. How old was she? How much longer did she live?

It's not so hard these days to find images of women with mastectomy scars. One of the most famous is the artist Matuschka's 1993 self portrait on the cover on *The New York Times Magazine*. We can imagine what the Frenchwoman looked like after her surgery, though radical mastectomies were more the norm back then than now.

In sixty-three years we went from one woman taking a picture of another woman's removed breasts, to a woman taking a picture of her own scarred self after her breast was cut away. *Beauty Out of Damage*, Matuschka called her self-portrait.

I wonder what Miller did with the breasts after she was finished with them. Who threw them away? I would bet they did not make it into a cemetery.

A dozen years later, Miller was photographing the European theater of war for *British Vogue*. In Saint Malo she accidentally stepped on the severed hand of an American soldier. She went on to photograph Buchenwald and Dachau; and in an extreme show of bad taste, in Munich she posed for a photo in Hitler's bathtub. This photo became infamous.

After the war she stowed her cameras and turned to cooking and drinking. She died in 1977, of cancer. I don't know what kind.

January 26. What Scar?...

...I asked Linc today. He'd asked me if I remembered showing everyone my scar last night. I thought it might have been the scar under my collarbone, a raised pink almond sliver where the port had been inserted and removed. It wasn't that scar. Apparently, under the influence of demon rum (or rather, tequila) I flashed my mastectomy scar twice. Were people horrified? I asked. He said no.

There were six of us at the table at Fernando's and a couple carafes of margaritas. Today Mitch reported that I kept asking him, Do you want to know a secret? but I told the same one or two over and over. I didn't ask him what I told him.

I hadn't been this drunk for about ten years. It made me realize why people drink, why frat boys have frat parties and people go to bars and sling back the beers. Because you get giddy and nothing matters and you're out of control.

And then you have patches of memory.

Did we have flan? I asked Mitch. We had. I remembered two shared dishes of flan and I remember ordering shrimp Veracruz and I remember the food coming but I don't remember eating it. Mitch said that his girlfriend Laurie told me that I didn't need reconstruction.

Alcohol unleashes inhibitions. Does this mean that I really want to show my scar? Perhaps. I was thinking of that Beauty Out of Damage photo and wondering if I should have a picture like that of myself on the cover of this book.

I'm usually the only one in the locker room at the park district building when I change for step aerobics. I've wondered what the reaction would be if someone saw me. I'm sharing a room with Miz P at an upcoming conference. I've imagined myself asking her if she'd like to see the scar. I think the scar is interesting. I've wanted to see friends' scars but thought it impolite to ask. I saw a mastectomy scar for the first time at the former Women's Gym, about twenty years ago. One of the proprietors had cancer and it seemed to me then that she came back to exercise a week after surgery. It couldn't have been that short a time, but it seemed like it. I was impressed that she'd returned so quickly. She's still fine, and teaching karate.

I read somewhere about a woman going topless at a swimming pool, so that you could see the scars from her double mastectomy. The other women complained. You must cover your breasts because they are sexual. Right? But if the breasts are erased, is their former site too sexual, too?

There's an odd new Canadian project on line sponsored by Schick and Rethink, a breast cancer charity. It's got the horribly coy title of Booby Wall, and it's picture after picture of women's breasts, sent in by the women themselves (supposedly). I saw two photos of the one-breast-and-scar combo, and one photo of reconstructed breasts without nipples. The campaign is to get women, especially young women, to Touch, Look and Check (TLC) their breasts. *Booby* connotes sniggering and disrespect. At least it does to me. How many idiots did it take to come up with this concept?

I will not be uploading pictures of my breast-and-scar. To see my chest, you'll have to come to the locker room. Or wait till I'm once-in-a-blue-moon drunk.

January 28. The Essential Guide

Little gray mice have come in from the extreme cold and we are trying to kill them. They're cute but they are home invaders, bringer of germs and worse, I tell myself. We've caught a couple of them in traps but there are more, running around the kitchen and office and laughing at us. The mice are wily. You can see why scientists use them all the time in experiments. I set a trap with Nutella and put it in the kitchen drawer that had mouse droppings. Nothing the next day, but less Nutella. I put a blue poison pellet on top and the pellet was gone. I wedged in a little piece of the pellet. That was gone too. Then I got some cheese and pushed it under this little vent on the plastic platform of the trap. This morning I checked and the trap was gone and there was blood about five inches away from where the trap had been. I figured we'd caught the mouse and Linc had thrown away the trap and mouse when he got up hours before.

For some reason I opened the drawer further. There was a mouse in the back it. His feet were caught in the trap. He looked at me with his big black eyes. He hopped around. I knew I had to kill him. I called Linc and he said he'd heard him jumping around but figured he'd die soon. Thanks a lot. He advised me to put the mouse and trap in a plastic bag and bang them against the concrete outside. But that involves getting dressed. I knew I had to put the mouse out of its misery.

First I covered him with cardboard—an empty cracker box that I flattened. I was thinking I should get a hammer to smoosh him with but then decided a big book would be better.

This was probably the first time I've used the *Chicago Manual of Style: The Essential Guide for Writers, Editors and Publishers, 14th edition.* I recommend it highly. This is definitely an instance when the spiral-bound *AP Stylebook*, which I refer to more often, would not have been as useful.

February 8. About the Bitches

I thought Susan Sontag showed everyone that our personality defects don't cause our cancer. Now we have the lovely bestselling Skinny Bitches telling us the opposite, and I would bet that more people have heard of them than the late Sontag. The authors of *Skinny Bitch: A no-nonsense, tough-love guide for savvy girls who want to stop eating crap and start looking fabulous* are counseling those savvy girls to go vegan and organic. Nothing wrong with that, except some of their science seems a bit loose. And then we get to page 189, where the Bitches praise, quote and paraphrase case studies from Dr. Carolyn Myss' book, *Anatomy of the Spirit*. To wit: *It is no coincidence that Julie was diagnosed with breast and ovarian cancer, reflecting her lack of self-love.... 'Joanna' was married to a man who had multiple affairs, which she knew about but tried to live with. Not surprisingly, she developed breast cancer.* But then she confronted her husband, left the marriage—and recovered! Of course!

The authors do say that they're not saying that everyone who's sick is responsible for bringing the illness upon him or herself. But that it's possible.

Thank you so much, Skinny Bitches, for blaming us.

I can't take this book back to the store because I didn't buy it. A co-worker of Linc's did. She had a lumpectomy and I guess is trying to clean up her act. We are all trying to. But the Skinny Bitches aren't the ones who should be directing us.

And they're not the only ones who think this way. Here's Sheryl Crow on CNN.com, verbatim: The idea that metaphysically the breasts represent nourishment and that there is a connection with breast disease and a lack of nourishment, whether it be allowing others to nourish or lack of self-nourishment, is one that strikes me. For me, it was a time of awakening to the idea that perhaps I had not allowed other people to take care of me but instead had always put everyone else and their needs before me and my needs.

February 20. Blut und Boden

So. I've got a new disease. Or condition. It's rare, and usually strikes men over sixty. Attentive readers will recall that I have too many platelets in my blood (aka essential thrombocythemia). I've found out I also have too many red blood cells. The official term is polycythemia vera. I have the non-hereditary gene mutation, JAK2, which is found in 95 percent of the people who have this. My hematologist (you know you're in trouble when you have a hematologist) told me yesterday I probably had it, and she looked at my blood results today and confirmed it. I make too many things, I said to the hematologist yesterday—starting with cancer, which is the production of too many cells in an uncontrolled way. She said, Yes, you make too many things. The first-line treatment for this, she told me, comes from the 13th century. Leeches? I asked. Not leeches, she said, but you get a phlebotomy. You go to LifeSource and get a pint taken out. You can't donate this pint because it's filled with too-thick blood. Where does it go? I asked. Probably into a biohazard bag and then to a landfill, she said. I thought of my blood seeping into the earth. *Blut und Boden.*

It seems a shame to waste this blood. To spill it. Sharon uses blood meal on her plants because it's rich in nitrogen. The web tells me that meal comes from dried blood, which comes from animal processing in slaughterhouses. I wonder if I could ask to keep my pint o' red and take it home, dry it, and sprinkle it in the front yard. So I will have more to offer our tulips and irises and columbine than just my sweat.

The plan is to give a pint on Tuesday (the first time I could get an appointment) and also two weeks later, then go to Fancy Hospital to get my blood tested, talk to the doctor, and probably have two more sessions two weeks apart. From there I would probably get my prophylactic phlebotomy every one, two or three months.

I need to rid myself of this thick blood because otherwise it maybe maybe maybe could cause blood clots, stroke, heart attack. I have learned what the signs of a blood clot are and that you can get an ultrasound to show if you have one. If this venesection, as the Brits call it, doesn't work, then there's Plan B, which involves chemotherapy. Mild. In the form of a pill called hydroxyurea.

My hematologist asked if I had itching. I said, mostly after taking a shower, and she said that's a symptom. I had noticed but I hadn't thought it meant anything. I also have hot flashes, which is not news to attentive blog readers or anyone who has been in a room with me lately. While flashing, my face and ears turn red. The doctor said that the phlebotomy might help with my hot flashes. So that's good news. (I keep thinking lobotomy and have to remind myself that one is brain and one is blood. No ice picks for Cancer Bitch.)

On the Internet you can send off for leeches of your own. They are non-returnable.

March 9. Hoisting a Pint or, the Annals of Polycythemia Vera (in Vera Veritas)

Two weeks ago I went to LifeSource and got a pint of blood removed. I go again on Tuesday. I think the blood-letting has helped. I may be getting less red in the face and sweating less upon exertion and upon hot-flashing.

The other morning I woke up to NPR and thought I heard that British veterans with my disease were suing the government. I figured it had to be part of my dream world, but it was real. Apparently hundreds of British and New Zealand servicemen witnessed nuclear tests in the South Pacific in the 1950s, and claim that the radiation exposure caused them to develop polycythemia and other illnesses. Some suffered immediate effects from the radiation: *Several chaps lost teeth, and others lost their hair,* according to a serviceman who was eighteen at the time and a radio operator aboard a ship. *So a lot of wives and sweethearts waited in Devonport to welcome back bald fiancés and bald boyfriends with a few teeth missing.*

Others developed PV later or cancers. Some 700 of them have banded together to sue the British Department of Defence for compensation.

The former radio operator quoted above was diagnosed with polycythemia in 1974. The BBC refers to it as a rare form of blood cancer that his doctors have linked to his exposure to radiation. (For his sake and the sake of the lawsuit, the disease should be as dire as possible; it's sometimes considered pre-cancerous, as a small percentage of people with it develop leukemia, and it's sometimes considered cancer, but it's not really cancer-cancer.)

I felt like saying, Aha, when I read about the British lawsuit, though I have never sailed the high seas for the United Kingdom. I'm of a mind to blame large institutions for bad things that happen to people. But I was never around a nuclear test. I had a lot of chest X-rays as a child because of my asthma and the two times I had pneumonia, but how could I ever prove a connection between the X-rays and the polycythemia? I'm not part of a group of sailors or soldiers or anything else that had repeated chest X-rays. I am a lone Cancer Bitch from the lone prairie. With extra-thick blood and a bad attitude.

March 19. I Was Marching

I'm not sure what my favorite color is or what my favorite breed of dog is (dachshunds some days, beagles, others) but I know what my favorite chant is. It's: Show me what democracy looks like. *This is what democracy looks like.* Tell me what democracy sounds like. *This is what democracy sounds like.*

I like it because it's accurate.

I am marching with the Code Pink women's group up Michigan Avenue, holding pink signs and banners aloft, and the shoppers and other pedestrians flanking us on the sidewalk are either neutral or making the V peace sign. The cops are out in force at bends in the road. At the foot of the Michigan Avenue bridge there were about sixty of them—a half dozen on horseback, a few with dogs, a lineup in riot gear, batons ready for action. But they didn't use them. This is not Mexico City or Paris or Chicago, 1968, or Tiananmen Square, 1989, or even Chicago 2003, when anti-war protesters were blocked and arrested en masse, and this is not Lhasa, Tibet. This is Chicago and we have a permit, we are orderly, most of us, though there are a few young men in front of me jumping and dancing haphazardly in a way that makes me think they're anarchists who wouldn't mind disturbing the peace. They are examples of what anthropologist Esther Newton has called her *enema man*. He is the person in your march who you are ashamed of, who does not represent you and your lovely well-behaved and acceptable self. She describes him in her book *Margaret Mead Made Me Gay*. It's 1971 and she's taking part in a gay pride march in New York City, though she's scared she'll be recognized. And then she sees a pale man with a sign that says, Pennsylvania Enema Society and he's carrying a disgusting enema bag, and she's even more self-conscious, that she'll be judged by association. But she writes: *But the revolution is less authentic for every oppressed person it excludes. The enema man is ... my forbidden self twisted into human flesh, just as I am the twisted flesh of the straight woman's forbidden self.*

The anarchists, the people who want to overthrow the government, who believe that Bush was behind 9/11, who want Israel to disappear, these are the people with unacceptable opinions, whom I don't want to be linked with, but who are part of the coalition against the war. I have chosen to be with them.

This is what democracy looks like, I'm telling the people on the sidelines. Maybe it's because I want them to like me. To understand that our country allows freedom of speech, that we are not unpatriotic or un-American, that we are exercising our First Amendment rights. We're all in this together, whether we agree or not. I am moved by these words, these thoughts, a little choke in my throat. So this is democracy and it's good and it feels good.

And marching is just one thing that a citizen does in a democracy. And I wonder: Are we making headway? Are we being heard where it counts? Are we stopping the war?

April 7. The Archivists

The Smart University archivists came by today to Cancer Bitch Central. They filled up one-and-a-half gray acid-free boxes, made from a flat pre-boxes. They took papers I wrote in college, syllabi from my student years and from my teaching (at the same place), some photographs (of a campus landmark, of a tiny park that's now fancily landscaped), satirical newspapers created by summer high school students on campus. It seems almost comical, these two guys ringing the bell and going through my papers. Taking what could be junk and treating it well. Or else it seems sinister. (I read too many accounts of Nazi soldiers coming into people's houses and rifling through belongings.) But I brought the archivists' visit on myself. Linc and I are thinking of moving, are moving toward moving, and I am a pack rat, and I have trouble throwing things away. I will pay $7 to send a box of taped interviews and papers to strangers (at the Tamiment Library at NYU, which I did earlier this year) but I cannot not throw out the same material. The archives at Smart University is always issuing e-mails to faculty, reminding us to save and send for posterity. (Its motto: When in doubt, *don't* throw it out.) So that is why I e-mailed them, offering my wares. I also offered my personal writerly papers, but the archives said I wasn't famous enough (said this nicely, of course, talking about limited space, etc., etc.). I felt some regret at letting my coursework go, but I can visit it whenever I want, during business hours. At least I can visit once the stuff is catalogued, and I can speed up that process by writing a bio and sending it in. The archivist told me to look at bios on its site for models. I have and I see that there was a prof who tried to enter Tibet in 1922. After being turned away, he sneaked in, dressed as a so-called Tibetan coolie, and then wrote a book, *To Lhasa in Disguise.* He is represented by five boxes of goods at the archives. As I read the bios of the other donors, I feel pretentious. There's no one else as young as I am, and I'm not young. But I had cancer and have a pre-cancerous blood disease. Part of my motivation is the possible imminence of my demise. I think: This will be one less task for Linc. Though it's just the tip. I still have six four-drawer file cabinets in my office at home. I have files and files of journal entries and accounts of my dreams (boring; but after toting them around for thirty years, I'm loath to throw them out) and letters and even faxes. I have my bat mitzvah speech and notes my friends passed to me in seventh grade, and comic strips I drew featuring talking French pastry, and research on the Weimar

Republic, back when you had to go through everything so painstakingly via newspaper indices and microfilm and -fiche.

My work will help future researchers who want to write on the history of journalism and liberal arts education. My papers will be catalogued and tucked away, not too far from the Leopold-Loeb ransom note and other treasures.

When I was at the University of Iowa Writers' Workshop, we were told that copies of all our stories and poems that we discussed in class were sent automatically to the university archive, the idea being that at least some of our peers would become famous. When I took anseminar on biography, we often talked about the surfeit of information. The problem of the future, we said, will be surplus—too many documents, too many photos, too many home videos. How will researchers be able to sift through and weigh? What will our family members, not yet born, appreciate having and what would they rather not be bothered with?

The other day I talked on the phone to my mother and she said she'd received so many nice notes from people who had attended her birthday festivities in March. Once a friend of hers told her that you keep notes and cards so you can read them in your old age. I'm in my old age now, my mother said, so I can throw them away.

April 22. Death

1. ... and Taxes

This year, my accountant asked me again if I saw the world any differently because of the cancer. I said no. Which is mostly true; I now have one more thing to worry about. As I grow older and possibly middle-aged I think that even if I lived to an old age, I could die relatively soon, in thirty-five years or so. That's fewer years than I've already been alive. To rephrase the coal-miners' song a bit, Another day older and deeper in death. Linc's mother is eighty-five and walks two miles every day and exercises in water and on land. My mother is eighty and walks in the mall and goes to her Jewish mothers' exercise class and to book club and to lectures and bridge games and has two or three theater subscriptions. She even drives at night.

Neither of them has had cancer.

2. An Accounting

But it would be disingenuous to say I haven't learned anything from this experience. This is what I have learned:

That you can switch oncologists.

That you can wait to get breast reconstruction; you don't have to have it right away.

That you can say you don't want medical fellows to check you out first in the fullness of their ineptitude.

That it's hard to tell which is worse, emotional or physical pain, because *in extremis* they come together.

That if they say your chemo will cause your hair to fall out, it will, even though your hair is thick and coarse.

That chemo doesn't have to cause nausea though it is ill-advised to eat meals rich in butter for a few days after a session.

That some people don't know how to react to a cancer diagnosis and will disappear.

That a person with whom you were friendly, who was there when you received the cancer phone call, will be decidedly unempathic and in the course of a year, will never ask how you are feeling.

That not everybody has a partner who responds like Linc—meaning that not everyone's partner will do what you take for granted: go to appointments with you and tell you to listen to your body and wonder if he's doing enough for you and be somewhat opposed to reconstruction.

That your sister will call you after every chemo.

That you can ask women with reconstructed breasts to show you their new breasts and they will, and they'll let you feel them, too.

That just because someone has had breast cancer doesn't mean you have anything in common ideologically, but you still have *something* in common.

That you will grow to hate pink ribbons because they represent a system that lets people feel good about being against breast cancer, and that doesn't question the causes of the epidemic.

That long after you feel fine you'll find yourself using breast cancer as an excuse: for being clumsy in aerobics, for being late to appointments, for all your failures.

That there is such a thing as chemo brain but you're still responsible to check your appointment book.

That a person just on the periphery of your life will unexpectedly bring you a very nice dinner.

That for you what's normal and even egotistical (writing about your experience) will seem to others to be courageous.

That some people will know that just sending a card is a very nice thing to do.

That people will offer to drive you to chemo when what you really want from them is time and talent to refresh your head decorations.

That you can take public transportation to and from chemo.

That the pharmacist can make a special thick potion to treat mouth sores.

That your bald and decorated head will make you feel special and defiant.

That jagua, made from the genipap fruit, is better than henna because it's darker. And that there's no such thing as black henna. What people call black henna is plain henna adulterated with hair dye, and it can cause skin lesions, scary photos of which you can find on the Internet.

That at some hospitals, people don't have to wait hours for chemo.

That just because your cancer-cousin in Marin County has huggy nurses and doctors and a view of Mount Tamalpais from the chemo rooms and organic popsicles in the hospital cafeteria, her port can still get infected, causing her to need daily treatment with antibiotics.

That even having had cancer, you will still have a hard time getting yourself to eat right and exercise.

That it's possible to teach a week after a mastectomy but it's not advisable.

That in hospitals they still wake you up to see how you're doing.

That you don't have a bad reaction to general anesthesia.

That the best thing anyone can say to someone with cancer is: So-and-so had it years ago and is doing great.

That a day before your surgery to get a breast removed from your body, someone who is normally sensitive will tell you about her breast reduction surgery, prefacing it by saying, You'll like this story, and you'll be too shy to tell her that the two operations are not the same.

That it's possible for the surgeon to remove only one lymph node in sentinel node surgery.

That you prefer medical care by women.

That even though breast cancer is an epidemic around these parts, the flatness over your heart will make you feel specially marked, like you're saying to people, See my wound, and you know you shouldn't use your surgery like that.

That you're glad to have had chemo as a precaution because you know someone who didn't and her cancer came back. And back.

That the reason for your cancer could be mosquito foggers or pesticides in the lawns of your youth or chest X-rays or hormones in the milk or air pollution and you'll probably never know.

Or maybe it's the water.

That eight months after chemo, people will still be saying, with surprise, how good you look, and you won't be sure if it's because they expected you to look bad. And you know that part of the reason you look healthy is because your pre-cancerous blood disease makes you flush.

That it's good you got hit at fifty-one instead of thirty-one or twenty-one; older patients have better prognoses. That now you know you handled your friend's sister's dire diagnosis all wrong years ago, saying, I'm sure she'll be fine, when she was, in effect, dying in her twenties.

(Don't think about people who died. Don't think about Beth or Judy or Harriet or Tootie or Laurie or Julie or Grace Paley.)

That some people with breast cancer don't like to talk about what stage they're in, because staging is too much like fate or destiny, and Susan Sontag had stage 4 in the 1970s, and with imported chemo, she lived another thirty years.

That the first time you read this list out loud, a sunny-side-up pediatric oncologist will ask you if you've always been so negative, and whether you've spent time with children with cancer, and what you learned from them, and you'll think of Jesse, and how happy everyone wasvwhen an adult friend discovered that he liked to have vanilla-scented lotion smoothed over his skin, it was a relief to be able to provide pleasure, and not feel so helpless. That's what you learned.

You have learned also that your eyelashes will come back but your eyebrows won't be as dark.

Maybe you will look back in twenty years and barely remember you had breast cancer or maybe it will kill you.

You don't know what will happen, how you will die, but you will die, even though you can't imagine the world going on without you.

Can it?

.

June 1. Postscript: Biting the Hand that Fed Me (Poison)

The morning was sunny and clear and mild today during the largest cancer survivors' celebration in the country. Of its kind. Meaning, this wasn't a pledge walk. About 3,600 people gathered in Grant Park downtown and then walked noncompetitively for four miles along the lakefront. Everyone seemed to be happily ambling along with friends and family, most wearing their designated T-shirts—purple for survivors, white for others. Just about everyone pinned a paper tag to their shirt back, having written the names of the people they were walking for. There was a man whose tag said, *my son Nolan*, and there was a kid next to him whose tag said, *ME!* A girl was walking between a man and a woman, whose tags read: *my sweet daughter Jam the champ!* And: *the most wonderful kid ever, Jam!* Others were *in memory: of Hozzie, of my grandma who died with cancer two years ago* (written in childish cursive), *my mother RIP 9-3-07, the 1,500 people that will die today!* There were about twenty-five people walking together for Roly Menendez, a twenty-five-year survivor. There were people with Team Madden caps and about thirty people walking near a flag with a photo of a woman named Nini Lyman on it. A man was herding them, calling them the Lymanettes, so he could take a group picture.

Nini was diagnosed with ovarian cancer in 1999 and died about two weeks ago.

A woman walking with perhaps an eleven-year-old girl was answering her questions. The woman said, Some don't make it and some do.

Along the way were banners with black-and-white head shots of smiling survivors, with their first names, kind of cancer, number of years of survival, and tired inspirational quotes:

A positive attitude is half the battle.

Now you can see how precious and vibrant life is through the eyes of a survivor. Never underestimate the healing power of a good laugh.

Some people get cancer and start dying—some people get cancer and start living. I think I started living.

I'm living proof that cancer is not a death sentence.

Next to one of the banners there stood the actual woman, a twenty-one-year ovarian cancer survivor. Two other women in purple were talking to her. One wore a turban. They discovered they had the same doctor. Isn't she wonderful? one of them said.

Along the way there were stations where you could get water and trinkets. Volunteers poured cups of water from plastic water jugs, others wore plastic hula skirts and handed out plastic leis. One person's spaniel got its legs caught in a lei. Walkers were handed free inflatable plastic beach balls and plastic mini-bottles of bubbles. Volunteers removed plastic stars-and-stripes maracas from individual plastic bags and gave them to the walkers. Emblazoned on each maraca was Abraxis BioScience, one of the walk's sponsors. You could also get a mint wrapped in red, white and blue and a tri-colored ribbon with a gold medal made of plastic.

The walk ended back where it started. There was music and good cheer. People lined up for sandwiches from Subway (Please ONLY Take ONE of Each Food Item. Thank You!) each in its own plastic bag, packets of Oreos and pretzels, apples and individual plastic bottles of water. Then they sat on the grass and watched performances by the Jesse White Tumblers and the Trinity Irish Dancers. Kids ran up and down an inflatable playground and jumped on an inflatable trampoline (after their parents had signed waivers). They could get temporary tattoos and take finger puppets, a miniature plastic ball-in-the-hole game and tiny boxes of clay. You could look at the Dedication Wall, where people had written messages: *To all families who lifes [sic] have been touch [sic] with cancer. May we continue to walk until God gives us a cure!*

Gramps, you'd love the twins! (and I know they'd love you.)
Thank you [Fancy] Hospital for giving me all these years!

After the dancers and a speaker, there was an official group photo of all the survivors in their purple shirts, and Cancer Bitch in her beige Breast Cancer Action Bad Girls of Cancer T-shirt, sitting on the front row, middle. I ordered a copy of the photo for $10. No one asked me about my shirt.

After the photographer finished, there were hugs and tears.

The walk was sponsored by the Fancy cancer department, and purple just happens to be the color of the university connected to Fancy. All of the head shots were of patients who had been treated at Fancy. I suppose other hospitals could have sponsored this walk, but they didn't. A cynical person might think that this event was created not for the survivors at all, but in order to be a 3,600-strong walking advertisement for cancer treatment at Fancy. (And why not? And maybe Fancy saved my life, too.)

I kept thinking about the plastic. Why O why was there so much? Used plastic is either incinerated or dumped in a landfill or (more rarely) gets new life as a deck or patio furniture. When some plastics are incinerated, they release dioxin, officially declared a carcinogen by the EPA. I don't know if any or all of these plastics are the kind that would release dioxin, or if how they will meet their end (or almost-end; it's hard to make plastic disappear) or if any contain the additive that behaves like estrogen. But I do know that the handouts could have been more eco-friendly. Two days after the walk, I asked a Fancy spokeswoman about the plastic and she said that she didn't know if the organizers had thought a lot about it, that they were just thinking of fun, economical things to give out. She said my point was really good. It's something we can look into, she said.

I went by myself to the celebration, registering when I got there, for $20, and I got a T-shirt, breakfast, lunch, water and the tchochkes. It was $15 if you pre-registered, and the event, the fifteenth in a row, is supposed to break even. I walked alone while writing, a cynical Cancer Bitch, while at the same time thinking that no one at Fancy Hospital had done anything to commemorate my last round of chemo, but that this event could be a way to mark it, communally. I thought about bringing all my chemo escorts together next year and having them walk by my side. I thought it might be meaningful. It might be festive.

Time Passed...

May 7, 2024. Seventeen Years After Breast Cancer

I've never returned to the Fancy Hospital march and celebration.

We bought a house. We live in it. I am alive. I forgot to say that. I am still unreconstructed. I've learned that an unreconstructed Southerner is one who has not accepted Reconstruction. A horrible thought. I interviewed people in the South. I came back. We painted the walls of the house yellow, orange, mint green, lilac. We did not paint it ourselves. We paid men to paint it. The house was built around 1890 and the first weeks I was mean to Linc because I thought I should make all the interior design decisions, that he had no right. We have a yard that people admire because Linc has planted poppies that he got from his mother in downstate Illinois. They take over the corner. I've counted sixty blooms at a time. They're coming early this year, a sign of global warming. Last summer in front we had tall purple aster, bright orange Mexican sunflowers, seven-foot-high yellow sunflowers. My friend Jennifer brought us the starts for the Mexican sunflowers. In her own yard in Ohio the deer eat hers up. Linc planted milkweed, mums, native roses. We plant begonias, pansies, marigolds, geraniums. We grow basil and cherry tomatoes and bitter kale and green onions in pots. We grow parsley, lots of parsley, for the black swallowtail butterflies. Sometimes I bring the caterpillars inside. They grow from small black worms to fat striped sybarites. In the fall we miss having something alive, alive, and eating, on the buffet in the living room.

Instead of down the alley we live half a mile west of Barry and Sharon. Sharon still drives to Indiana to teach. Barry had a stroke and can't move much more than part of an arm. He has round-the-clock care, at home. He talks very softly. His voice is better in the morning, better when he takes sips of water. For a while he was dictating poems to undergraduates to transcribe and send to literary magazines. Seth, their son, the Neighbor Boy, met a lovely woman in New Orleans, married her, and they moved to Texas.

People I know who had breast cancer have died: Elyse, diagnosed around the same time I was. Sonia, diagnosed after. My therapist. (At the funeral I found out I wasn't the only client who made her laugh uproariously. We all did.) My student Nicole, who did standup toward the end.

Two aunts and two uncles died. Two local one-breasteds are still alive. Cousins have died, cousins have been born. A friend with my same stage of cancer died years ago. My polycythemia vera caused terrible itching but it's under control with a very expensive chemo tablet. When I was going through breast-cancer treatment, I mostly considered PV to be pre-cancer. Since, I've called it cancer. There's a reason for that. The US National Heart, Lung, and Blood Institute website: *Once considered a blood disorder only, polycythemia vera is now defined as a rare, chronic blood disorder that is a type of cancer.* So that means I'm still Cancer Bitch. My PV is indolent, as am I.

Linc has retired and works part time writing, he volunteers working to combat climate change. I am no longer at Smart U. My forty-plus-year love-hate relationship with the university is over. Perhaps. I edit for private clients. I run a literary magazine. I discovered I love to pull weeds. I travel around talking about my writing, and sometimes cancer.

Amelia had breast cancer. She and I shared a few meals. We don't know how to get closer. We bang against one another's rough edges. The skin where my breast used to be still itches. My mother had a lumpectomy, outpatient, when she was eighty-six. Now she's ninety-six and driving, reading, playing bridge, going to the ballet. She survived Hurricane Harvey. She survived COVID in 2023. I've had COVID, the flu, I come down with bronchitis once or twice a year. I'm just getting over human metapneumovirus, which I thought was pneumonia but isn't. My allergists' office is always so attentive when I'm sick that I send them chocolates and bread. The last time, the Fellow took all the treats home. He's a starving student, the physician assistant said.

When George Floyd was brutally murdered by the state, institutions suddenly discovered they'd been ignoring white supremacy. As an adjunct at Brain Trust University, non-credit division, I went to meetings to discuss curriculum change, to find ways to make race relevant when discussing the classics. Changes were made. A year after treatment I joined a rowing group for breast cancer survivors. I was a terrible rower without a sense of rhythm or memory of what to do when. I rowed for nine years until my heels hurt too much—from walking—to continue. We rowed in polluted water where condoms and tampons and shit bobbed along the top after a storm. There were women who had mets—metastasis—who were strong rowers, who were athletes. Women who were dying who were so much better rowers than I, though you're not supposed to compare, and everything isn't supposed to revolve around me. But if not me, then who? Who else is there to sing the song of myself?

During the pandemic Linc and I started walking at night, four miles, five, more. I discovered the river was only two miles away. We stir-fried vegetables every night. I made bread. I lost weight. I think every so often about getting a breast replacement but the thought of pain and long recovery stops me. I'm still making bread. I'm writing short stories set in Europe. We still walk.

A friend dyed her hair blue when her granddaughter did. I started dyeing mine red and purple. Semi-permanent, and I don't look up the ingredients to see if they're carcinogenic. I feel young. I'm not. For a long time people older than I ran things and now they're all younger. Three kinds of bees come to the front yard, and monarch butterflies. We liked the idea of them supping on Mexican sunflowers before their flight down to Mexico. Problems everywhere are intractable. I don't have to list them for you. Last time there was a big snow I made a dachshund and a snowman holding a leash.

They tell me I'm not middle-aged any more.

NPR's Scott Simon interviewed me and asked if cancer books have to be funny.

I don't know.

I'm not telling you everything. I never can or will. Cafés have shut down: Café Avanti, Emerald City in Lakeview. Kopi is still around. Women & Children First bookstore is thriving.

I finally read Audre Lorde's *The Cancer Journals*. She writes of going to the doctor's office to get her stitches removed. In the waiting room the nurse admonishes her for not wearing the lambswool puff that's supposed to temporarily fill in for the breast that was removed. She tells Lorde that the obviousness of her missing breast is *bad for the morale of the office.*

Lorde is outraged, writing that prostheses are usually functional. Think of dentures, artificial limbs. *Only false breasts are designed for appearances only.* She mentions the celebrated Israeli general Moshe Dayan, famous for his eyepatch, a souvenir of war: *Nobody tells him that he is to go get a glass eye, or that he is bad for the morale of the office. The world sees him as a warrior with an honorable wound.*

Lorde writes that her own scars *are an honorable reminder that I may be a casualty in the cosmic war against radiation, animal fat, air pollution, McDonald's hamburgers and Red Dye No. 2, but the fight is till going on, and I am still a part of it. I refuse to have my scars hidden or trivialized behind lambswool or silicone gel.*

That she uses Dayan as an example is astounding. I have to agree that he lost his eye in a noble cause—he was fighting against Vichy forces in 1941.

I wear a prosthesis for formal occasions—weddings, any gathering where my mother is present. Insurance paid for the squishy fake breast, though I had to throw in $45 more for a stick-on nipple
I get mammograms yearly. What I've done more of since cancer: travel. Sofia, Bulgaria; Belgrade, Serbia; Wroclaw, Poland; Berlin; Vienna; London—for conferences. Paris, because it's Paris. The American South, for research: Selma, where my great-grandparents came after leaving Lithuania; Jackson; then Laurel, Mississippi, where my father was born.
I found out about a race rebellion in Houston in 1917, which we didn't learn about in school. I read 5,000 pages of court martial testimony and wrote a play. I'm not a playwright. It might become something else.
I buy yahrzeit candles. I meditate weekly with a group from Gilda's Club. These people have died: Paula, Sara, David, Lynette, Laura, Erica, Linc's mother and aunt and uncle. I helped—barely—with my high school reunion; the names of our dead kept growing on the website. Linc washed all our sweaters and they shrank. I washed some in baby shampoo to reshape them. It almost worked. Papers still pile up in my office. I'm working on my French. I have seven tall file cabinets. I collect discarded grocery lists. I like paper. I donated two scrapbooks to an archive. Re-reading this book I realized I never gave more information to the genetic counselor. We have two great-nephews and grandchildren. Two of them asked me, hesitating, why I had only one breast. I forgot the word they used. I told them it was OK to ask. I told them I'd had cancer. They were surprised. We (Linc) fight against the planet growing hotter. The evidence keep piling up against fossil fuels: besides heating the planet, they're linked more and more to cancers and other disease, more and more often affecting people in marginalized communities. I suggest that seeking out information on these risks (see bcpp.org) is more helpful than putting on pink clothes and walking from city to city because you're against breast cancer. I mean, who's *for* it, except other breast cancer cells? Linc does the boring work of fighting climate change by going to meetings and organizing and lobbying to change laws, while other people, good people, wring their hands. I understand that. It feels good to wring your hands, especially when you do it so hard that it hurts, just a little.

May 28, 2024. Notes on Asymmetry

After this book was first published, people asked me whether I'd had reconstruction. Apparently I'd left readers hanging. Other people would ask me to my face; they would ask me to my chest: Did you have surgery? They couldn't all have ocular problems, the kind where straight lines look wavy or vice versa. They knew. They could tell. They just wanted confirmation. Maybe they were really asking, Why didn't you? Can't you tell you're lopsided?

Or they were saying, You should. You really should. Just go back to the hospital and get a new one to replace the old.

That's what Americans do, right? Our capitalist system is based on planned obsolescence. Your original left breast had flaws. They cut it off and threw it away, probably burned it. So get a new one. Insurance pays for it.

Insurance even pays for the other breast to get a facelift so that it matches the new one.

Early on, when I met with plastic surgeons, they asked me what cup size I wanted. I didn't and don't think in cup sizes. Sometimes I would wear a 34 or 36 A and sometimes a B. I think men think that women think in cup sizes. Or maybe it's just me who doesn't have a clear idea how big an A or B is. All I ever wanted from a bra was a good fit that would cut the jiggle that hurt when I ran or jumped. Men also think that women want larger breasts than they truly do. Surgeons operate on women who are lying down so the new breasts seem smaller. You would think that doctors would know this. It's elementary physics. I've read accounts of women who told the surgeon how large they wanted their breasts to be, and woke up to the horror of their surgeon's generosity. Honey, you asked for a B but I gave you a D, because men know what girls really want.

If I hadn't had a partner when I was diagnosed, maybe I would have had reconstruction. Or maybe I would have worn my prosthesis more often. Or at least in winter. The thing is hot and sweaty in warm weather and you have to buy a special bra at a special bra store to hold the fake breast in place. The prosthesis is a funny thing. When you hold it, it does feel like a breast, it's soft and squishy.

I lost twenty-three pounds since COVID. Walked more, ate better. I now weigh the exact number of pounds that I've been listing for decades on my driver's license. I've thought for a long time that the people who work in the DMV are so dour because all day long people lie to them about their weight. I weigh more or less what I did when I met Linc, except I was two inches taller and I had a second breast. How much did that weigh? The prosthesis weighs 6.6 ounces. I just weighed my right breast by holding it on top of the platform of my digital postal scale: 1.9 pounds.

Most of the time I forget I don't have two breasts. Or I forget that I'm supposed to have two. One seems enough. I usually think I look elegant even if I'm wearing raggedy shorts and an old T-shirt and I'm taken aback by the reflection in a shop window of an untidy person with wild hair. Is that really me?

Because of skin-sparing surgery, I do have a little mound. I even noticed cleavage in one recent photo. I've never sought cleavage, not even toe cleavage, which people used to talk about fifteen or so years ago. For those who don't remember or who weren't paying attention, toe cleavage is when the front top of your shoe is so narrow that you can see the beginnings of your big toe and second toe. That line between the toes is the cleavage. It could also be the "crack" between two other toes. Does it turn men on? Shoe designer Christian Laboutin calls it a "second décolleté" in a 2006 article in the *Independent*. "A good shoe is one that doesn't dress you but undresses you." As a teen he hung out at the Folies Bergère and Moulin Rouge.

Enough about showgirls and shoegirls.

Celebrities who've gone flat: Kathy Bates, Anjelica Huston, Tig Notaro.

Being half-flat makes me feel like an intellectual, a being who rises above appearance. But if I don't care how I look, why do I brush mascara on my eyebrows that never grew back all the way after chemo?

Why do I feel smug when people complain about the look and feel of post-mastectomy breasts—and the tightness at the site when abdominal fat is used to form the breast; pain; a breast that doesn't have a good shape; the feeling from implants that something is inside you. Why do I note silently that implants need to be replaced after ten or twenty years? In addition, the silicone can escape from its sac and cause pain and hard lumps. Do I have to focus on the down side of reconstruction in order to convince myself that I made the right decision?

Audre Lorde: "[C]ertain other people feel better with that lump stuck into my bra, because they do not have to deal with me nor themselves in terms of mortality nor in terms of difference."

This is what breast cancer looks like.

We shed the old, the unnecessary: baby teeth; hair; finger- and toenails.
Cut them off.
Hymie the Jewish Tooth Fairy was the character who collected our teeth from under our pillows. He wrote, *Dear Sandy, Thanks for the excellent merchandise. I turn the teeth into beautiful pearls.*
I have lost grandparents, a father, lovers, a little gold ring my grandmother gave me with a heart holding my birthstone, friends, two red blouses, rain pants, a pair of sandals. I have lost shoelaces, heels, earrings, a lapis necklace. People lose blood, courage, joie de vivre. There is loss of wages, of country, of language, of domicile; loss of the imagined future, loss of the castle you built in the sky. The little tin soldier loved the dancer because he couldn't see the leg that was raised in arabesque.
I lost my breast and all I got is this lousy pink ribbon churned out by a factory and which symbolizes a corporation's desire to be seen as benevolent.

Top surgery removes an excess. Takes away that which is unwelcome in a female body inhabited by a male. Top surgery is the language of gain, it removes what hinders.
Appendectomy. Hysterectomy. Clitoridectomy.
Cephalectomy is removal of the head.
Hysteric-ectomy is removal of the hysteric.
We replace, implant, plump up, reshape, recover, reupholster.

Do I regret not getting an implant installed or having a trickier operation using my own body fat? Yes, no, yes, no. Years ago I heard about a trial lawyer who said she had to have reconstruction because appearance counted in her work, and by her work she really meant her sexiness. Her sense of herself, that she's no one if she's not sexy. What does "sexy" mean? That people want to have sex with her? That they're more interested in what she says because she's attractive, fuckable?
What are we supposed to be? Who do we want to be? Who are we?

My right breast is aware that her twin has gone, flown the coop. But she thinks only of herself, her horizontal scar above the nipple, from a biopsy, benign. The breast is a dumb creature. My left breast didn't know that the farewell party was for her. The breast wasn't doing much. Not being used except to fill out clothes, to receive touch, enjoy touch. To participate in symmetry. Not engaging in feeding a new generation.
Under my scars my skin itches. I can't reach the itch. It prickles underneath.
My breast was a part of me.
It is apart of me.

A surgeon cuts—into, around through, off, across. The surgeon is a master of prepositions. I say master because most surgeons are male, though mine wasn't.

I want a tank top that is open on the left side so that you can see the scars. I keep thinking that I will bare that side during the next Pride march, which is the closest we get to Bacchanal in Chicago, at least in my neighborhood. Exposing my non-breast is legal, because nipples are what make breasts obscene. This is illogical, because the nipple is the most hard-working, useful part.

I want to go to the henna place and get designs that cover all that non-breast area. I want people to notice. Why do I need that? Do I always have to be noticed? Admired for being different? I am original. Therefore—therefore, I deserve to live.

I was jittery one day last week and I said to Linc, Do you ever feel that you are bad, that you did something wrong, that everything about you is wrong? I was thinking *shame* but I didn't say it. He said, No. He does not question his right to exist.

What if I went around showing my left chest? I asked him. It would not be in good taste, he said. Unnecessary. This, he emphasizes, is only his opinion. He does not give or withhold permission. Why would I do it? Because I want to show people that a mastectomy is not a terrible thing. That you can play with it. You can play with cancer. That's one way of beating it. Refusing to despair. It is one way of being alive.

If I were a cicada, I'd be dead by now.

Breast Cancer Resources

African American Breast Cancer Alliance, www.aabcainc.org, programs and resources for Black women and men diagnosed with breast cancer, as well as their caregivers

American Association for Cancer Research, www.aacr.org, advocacy for research and education; on disparities in treatment: cancerprogressreport.aacr.org

Breast Cancer Action, bcaction.org, information on environmental causes of breast cancer, pinkwashing, breast cancer and fossil fuels (The organization closes December 2024.)

Breastcancer.org, guidance for people diagnosed with breast cancer, virtual meetups, info on clinical trials, en español

Breast Cancer Prevention Partners, www.bcpp.org, info and action to take on toxic chemicals and breast cancer

Cancer Support Community, www.cancersupportcommunity.org, links to support organizations around the country, including Gilda's Clubs, which provide classes, support, help line and information for cancer patients and caregivers, en español

Centers for Disease Control and Prevention National Breast and Cervical Cancer Early Prevention Program, www.cdc.gov/breast-cervical-cancer-screening, free and low-cost screenings

Earth Day, www.earthday.org, information on environment and climate and action you can take; report on plastic and health

Environmental Working Group, www.ewg.org, consumer guides on health dangers--including endocrine disruptors--in food and consumer products, en español

Equal Hope, www.equalhope.org, formerly Metropolitan Chicago Breast Cancer Task Force, free breast and cervical cancer screenings, reports on disparities in cancer care; en español

Johns Hopkins Health Library, www.johnshopkinshealth care.staywellsolutionsonline.com, info on drug interactions, efficacy of herbs and supplements, conditions and treatments

Living Beyond Breast Cancer, www.lbbc.org, information, support groups, help line, funding and funding resources, en español

National Breast Cancer Foundation, www.nationalbreastcancer.org, information and resources, support groups, retreats for metastatic patients, en español

Susan G. Komen, www.komen.org, helpline in English y español, resources including links to college scholarships for survivors; I've been hard on the organization in this book, but over the years it's improved, paying more attention to metastatic survivors and health disparities. It also provides financial assistance up to $400 to eligible people with breast cancer.

Tower Cancer Research Foundation Magnolia House, www.towercancer.org/tower-cancer-magnolia-house-classes, virtual wellness classes

About the Bitch

My friends say I shouldn't have called myself Cancer Bitch because, they say, I am not now and was not ever a bitch during surgery and chemo. But I thought it should be Cancer Something, and Babe was too young and Vixen was already taken. So I became the Bitch.

This chronicle is as true as I could make it. I haven't made anything up. A few names of individuals and their identifying characteristics were changed in the interest of privacy. There are no composite characters. The names of the coffee houses were not changed because they are independent and need the business.

No animals were harmed in the production of this book except a few mice, and they were home invaders.

For the 2024 paperback edition, I've edited the 2009 clothbound edition and have made some additions.

Notes and Updates

FIRST YEAR

January 16: To sit *shiva* means to literally sit on low stools in the home for seven (*shiva* in Hebrew) days, receive visitors, and recite the mourner's prayer twice a day.

January 24: A year and a half later, after a routine mammogram, I met with an attending radiologist who interpreted the new film for me. (There were calcifications, which were probably benign; come back in six months.) I told her that when I was first diagnosed, I had a bad experience with the Cold Blonde fellow, who hadn't called me when she said she would, and then when she did call, just said, It's positive, and seemed very cold. The radiologist looked in her records to see who that fellow was, said she was now out of state, and that she was sorry. She added that some patients might not even know what positive meant, they might have thought that it meant good news. She said she didn't like having people receive the news over the phone because you don't know where they are, and that it's really bad when you give the news to an elderly woman who's alone. I asked what training the fellows get and said that they should get better training, and she said the best thing is to give feedback, that's the only way they know if anything's wrong. I guess I should have said something at the time, but there was so much else going on. I was still teary about this. I hated that Cold Blonde.
    And I know that she was nervous, and aloof-seeming because she was nervous, and also seemed defensive, because she wanted to prove she was a Real Doctor while the patients were thinking she wasn't real and bona fide yet. And maybe it didn't help that she was pretty and blonde and maybe all her life had been trying to convince people that she really was smart.
    I think now I would be able to tell people they had cancer, but I wouldn't have been able to when I was younger. Why should some twenty-five-year-old know how to do it? I think the radiologists make the fellows do it because they don't want to. At a medical humanities conference I heard a med student (widow of a man who died of cancer in his twenties) talk about how her fellow med students would giggle when they were role-playing and taking turns delivering bad news. And she didn't want to chide them and tell them that it wasn't a laughing matter, she just let it go. I think the radiologists need to train the fellows how to talk to patients. What

makes this tricky is that you have to be secure if you're going to address the patient without pretense, and the teaching docs can't teach security, they can only encourage it. If you're secure, then you don't have to be absorbed in proving your expertise. You can pay attention to the needs of your patient.
Mishugas is Yiddish for craziness.

January 27: Komen has changed, a result of time and outside criticism. Its website emphasizes research and help for women with breast cancer and its mission to end breast cancer. Its city-to-city walks are now called "MORE THAN PINK WALK®"s. It provides financial assistance for those with breast cancer, too. It's now called Susan G. Komen ®.

January 31: *Les seins, ce sont moi* means *The breasts, they are me*, a riff on Gustave Flaubert's alleged quote about his most famous character: *"Madame Bovary, c'est moi."*

February 3: Regarding the wording "if I die "—There's a commercial for life insurance on the radio in which the announcer says you get the money if you don't die.

February 4: Your garden-variety American Jew is Ashkenazi; we make up more than 90 percent of the Jewish population in the US, with forebears from central, eastern, and western Europe, often Yiddish speakers. Most of the other 10 percent are Sephardic Jews originally from Spain (before the Inquisition) who traditionally speak Ladino (Judeo-Spanish). There are also Mizrahi Jews from the Middle East.

February 7: More than a year later, Cancer Bitch and Amelia effected a détente, and then a warming, and then a wall fell down. Amelia objected to the word "bitter" in this description but otherwise agreed with my characterization of our relationship and place in life. As of 2024, we haven't purposely gotten together in years. Are we missing out?

February 9: The *aleph-bais* is the Hebrew alphabet, named after the first two letters. It has various spellings. I'm being tricky here, because *"bais"* is the Yiddish pronunciation of the second letter. In Hebrew it's *"bet."* *"Aleph-bais"* evokes for me the Jew in the diaspora learning the ancient language from another land.

February 11: Barbara Ehrenreich's essay "Welcome to Cancerland" appeared in the November 2001 issue of *Harper's* magazine and was reprinted in *Best American Essays*. It later became part of her 2009 book *Bright-sided: How the Relentless Promotion of Positive Thinking Has Undermined America* (Metropolitan Books). She died in 2022 at eighty-one, after a stroke.

More February 11: Journalist Rose Kushner, one of the first women to write and publish candidly about her breast cancer, challenged the Halsted procedure because it automatically removed the breast, the underarm lymph nodes and both chest wall muscles. She also advocated for waiting between a biopsy and surgery. In her 1975 book, *Breast Cancer: A Personal History & an Investigative Report* (Houghton Mifflin Harcourt Press) she recounts her fight to find a doctor to perform the modified procedure that is common today. She died of breast cancer in 1990, at age sixty. Another Ashkenazi Jew. I consider her the first American breast cancer activist. She was an educator, resource provider and advocate. A good bio is at https://jwa.org/encyclopedia/article/kushner-rose .

March 20: In her essay, "Women and Honor: Some Notes on Lying," Adrienne Rich writes: "We have been expected to lie with our bodies: to bleach, redden, unkink or curl our hair, pluck eyebrows, shave armpits, wear padding in various places or lace ourselves, take little steps, glaze finger and toe nails, wear clothes that emphasized our helplessness." She first read the essay aloud at the Hartwick Women Writers' Workshop in June 1971. It was published as a pamphlet by Motheroot Press in Pittsburgh, 1977; reprinted in *Heresies: A Feminist Magazine of Art and Politics*, vol. 1, no. 1; and can be found in her collection, *On Lies, Secrets, and Silence: Selected Prose 1966-1979*, in various editions.

March 25: The information about AstraZeneca is from Samantha King's *Pink Ribbons, Inc.: Breast Cancer and the Politics of Philanthropy* (University of Minnesota Press, 2006), but it has been reported relatively widely elsewhere.

March 26: The Passover seder is the holiday dinner, which is served in a particular order, accompanied by particular prayers and the recounting of the story of Exodus. Seder is Hebrew for "order." The Haggadah is the book you read from. It means "telling."

April 2: Then Jewish Theological Seminary Chancellor Ismar Schorsh wrote on June 16, 2001, "Archaeology offers not the slightest confirmation of the biblical narrative [of the Exodus], only an abundance of evidence for its implausibility." He concludes: "Effective ritual has the power to transcend its origins and absorb new meanings." I found his commentary on *Parashah Sh'lakh L'kha*, Numbers 13:1–15:41 on the JTS website but haven't been able to refind it.

April 4: Reconstructionist Judaism was founded in the 1920s by Rabbi Mordechai Kaplan, who saw Judaism as an evolving civilization, and who tried to incorporate American democratic values into the practice of the religion. Reconstructionist Jews value ritual but don't believe that God made Jews the chosen people. OK, let's just say that Reconstructionist Jews are more likely to be vegetarians and wear Birkenstocks than other Jews are. And here's this joke: At an Orthodox wedding, the rabbi's wife is pregnant; at a Conservative wedding, the rabbi is pregnant; at a Reform wedding, the bride is pregnant; at a Reconstructionist wedding, both brides are pregnant. But back when our family Haggadah was published, Reconstructionism was mostly an offshoot of the Conservative movement. Back then, the Reform Jews were more liberal, but stuffy.

Dayenu is the title of and chorus of a thousand-year-old Passover song. It means "That would have been enough."

April 9: Information about the difference in breast cancer mortality between white and black women in Chicago is from the exhaustive article by Shane Tritsch, "The Deadly Difference," *Chicago Magazine*, October 2007. As of 2024, I could still locate it online. https://www.chicagomag.com/chicago-magazine/october-2007/the-deadly-difference/ On race and breast cancer, you can find Gray, J.M., Rasanayagam, S., Engel, C. *et al.* "State of the evidence 2017: an update on the connection between breast cancer and the environment" in *Environmental Health* 16, 94 (2017). https://doi.org/10.1186/s12940-017-0287-4, which states, "Racial and ethnic minorities often are exposed to disproportionately high levels and varieties of environmental pollutants in the U.S., as are people living in poverty. There are racial/ethnic differences in the body burden of different environmental chemicals that have been associated with increased risk for breast cancer. Blacks have higher body burden levels than whites or Mexican Americans of many chemicals including many polychlorinated biphenyls (PCBs), mercury, polyaromatic hydrocarbons (PAHs), and phthalates. Mexican Americans have higher levels of the pesticide dichlorodiphenyltrichloroethane (DDT). Varying body burdens of some chemicals including bisphenol A (BPA), polyfluorinated chemicals (PFCs) and triclosan, all commonly found in household products, are associated with both race/ethnicity and socioeconomic status. Yet ... socioeconomic status and race/ethnicity most probably serve independently as markers for other activities or circumstances that influence the level of exposures to potentially toxic chemicals." The Breast Cancer Research Foundation reports that Black women have more risk factors for breast cancer: obesity, diabetes, heart disease, and smaller likelihood of breastfeeding. "They are more likely than white women to have inadequate health insurance or access to health care facilities." As well, "Black women are disproportionately affected by more aggressive subtypes, such as triple-negative breast cancer (TNBC) and inflammatory breast cancer, and they are more likely to be diagnosed at younger ages and at more advanced stages of the disease." However, BCRF also found that there were *not* survival disparities between white women and other groups in states with expanded Medicaid after the Affordable Care Act. More at https://www.bcrf.org

May 14: On the $2.4 million study on prayer and healing, see "Study of the Therapeutic Effects of Intercessory Prayer (step) in cardiac bypass patients: A multicenter randomized trial of uncertainty and certainty of receiving intercessory prayer" in the *American Heart Journal* 151(4):934–942, April 2006. The study concluded: "Intercessory prayer itself had no effect on complication-free recovery from CABG, but certainty of receiving intercessory prayer was associated with a higher incidence of complications." Abilene Christian University biologist Savannah Vincent read studies going back to 1872 and concluded, in "Livin' on a Prayer: An Analysis of Intercessory Prayer Studies": "These studies are often either inconclusive or have varying results when compared to similar studies." She was writing in ACU's *Dialogue & Nexus*, Fall 2015-Spring 2016, Volume 3. This is a small publication, but I've read a number of studies on this topic and found problems with their set-up—either their populations were too specific or too small or the conclusions very subtle.

June 24: Marjorie Gross's essay "Cancer Becomes Me" originally appeared in the April 15, 1996, *New Yorker* and was reprinted in *Surviving Crisis: Twenty Prominent Authors Write about Events that Shaped Their Lives*, edited by Lee Gutkind (Tarcher/Putnam, 1997). Gross, a lead writer for *Seinfeld*, died of ovarian cancer on June 7, 1996, at the age of forty. Meanwhile, Dilbert was canceled in 2023 after creator Scott Adams made racist comments.

July 23: Since the first edition of this book was published, Naomi Wolf has become a conspiracist. Naomi Klein has written about the way people have conflated the two public Naomis in her 2023 book *Doppelganger: A Trip Into the Mirror World* (Farrar, Straus and Giroux).

August 13: The Woody Allen quote is, of course, from his book, *Without Feathers* (Ballantine, 1986). In 2009, we didn't know what we do now about him.

September 8: Watts Towers are outlandish, Outsider Art sculptures by the self-taught Simon Rodia, made between 1921 and 1955 out of steel pipes, mesh, mortar, sea shells, broken glass, and pottery. I hope to see them one day.

September 21: *Bikram* yoga, originated by Bikram Choudhury, is made up of specific Hatha yoga poses performed in a room heated to 105 degrees. I have not tried it; I carry my Bikramness with me. In 2023 the *Vancouver Sun* and *Yoga Journal* reported on allegations of sexual misconduct against him as well as civil suits in the U.S.

As of 2024, my hot flashes are caused by my polycythemia vera, and no longer by menopause or post-menopause, which one doctor told me are the same thing, which is the closest I'll get to time travel.

October 1: Later I ran into this young person, Jonah, again and invited him to our Torah study. He didn't join us. We were mostly amateurs and he grew up Orthodox and was very knowledgeable. By the spring he had a beard; he'd been taking testosterone. He moved on from our congregation to one that met more regularly, was more traditional. A few years later I read that Jonah had been hoping to become the foster parent of a troubled teen who tried to drown himself in Lake Michigan. Jonah tried to save him and in the process, drowned. This is sad on many levels. Jonah was about to turn twenty-eight. A kayaker found his body and tried CPR, but it was too late. I don't know what happened to the boy.

November 26: *Glatt* kosher is, informally, strict kosher. But it's not so simple. *Glatt* means "smooth" in Yiddish, and for an animal to be *glatt*, it must have smooth lungs without adhesions.

If the (dead) animal is found to have had unhealthy lungs, the whole carcass is considered nonkosher. At least by those who have *glatt* standards.

Dec. 2: I wrote that I didn't know how many people opt for reconstruction. It used to be that surgeons didn't consider reconstruction. Now some surgeons are resistant to patients who want to "go flat." According to the 2023 article "Going Flat: Mastectomy without Breast Reconstruction" in *Plastic and Reconstructive Surgery*, Sept. 2023, volune 152, issue 3, one-fifth of women felt their surgeons were pressuring them to have reconstructive surgery. What's striking is that the article authors say that a role of reconstruction "is to restore the form and function of tissue affected by cancer and associated treatments." Function? As Audrey Lorde points out, you can't feed a baby with reconstructed breasts. Maybe they're referring to function as experienced by a sexual partner. Authors are Kandi Lyndsay, Dr. Nellie Movtchan, Andrew Hostler, Dr. Michael Howard, and Chad Teven.

They quote another study, "Patient reported outcome measures (PROMs) following mastectomy with breast reconstruction or without reconstruction: a systematic review" in *Gland Surgery*, 2019, 8: 441-451. That article was a review of forty-two studies in English and Portuguese (because one of the authors was fluent in it). It showed that women who had reconstruction were more satisfied with their breasts than women who didn't have the plastic surgery. I mean, if you don't have a breast, how can you be satisfied with it? Women who had reconstruction had a somewhat higher level of pyschosocial well-being than those without the plastic surgery, about the same physical well-being, and a higher sexual well-being (55 points for reconstructed women vs. 44 points.) However, as we know, time changes all things: "As time passes, reduction in breast satisfaction is seen with all types of reconstruction options, with gluteal and thigh flaps having the worst long-term outlook..... In contrast, patients who opt to undergo mastectomy alone show an overall increase in reported breast satisfaction over time." Authors are surgeons Leonardo Z. Cordova, David J. Hunter-Smith, and Warren M. Rozen. I realize these studies don't give numbers on the percentage of women who choose reconstruction.

December 9: Donald Hall's now-classic and white-male-centric essay, "Poetry and Ambition," was delivered as the keynote speech at the Association of Writing Programs' annual conference in 1982, and was published in the *AWP Newsletter*, February/March 1987. It appears in Halls' collection, *Poetry and Ambition: Essays 1982–88* (University of Michigan Press, 1988). You can find it at https://poets.org/text/poetry-and-ambitionon Poets.org.

SECOND YEAR

January 1: Walter Benjamin writes in "Theses on the Philosophy of History" in *Illuminations*, edited and with an introduction by Hannah Arendt, translated by Harry Zohn (Schocken Books, 1968), that the Angel of History's "face is turned toward the past. Where we perceive a chain of events, he sees one single catastrophe which keeps piling wreckage upon wreckage and hurls it in front of his feet." The essay was first published in 1940.

January 4: From the University of Pittsburgh's Graduate School of Public Health, November 4, 2007, quoted on cancerprevention society.org

January 16: The study on fish ingesting Prozac and its ilk is "Analysis of paroxetine, fluoxetine and norfluoxetine in fish tissues using pressurized liquid extraction, mixed mode solid phase extraction cleanup and liquid chromatography–tandem mass spectrometry" (Try to ingest that title!) in the *Journal of Chromatography A*, Vol. 1163, Issues 1–2, 7 September 2007. Authors are Shaogang Chua and Chris D. Metcalfe.

January 20: See the January 17, 2008, *The New York Times* in the Skin Deep column in the Fashion & Style (!) section, "Do My Breast Implants Have a Warranty?" by Natasha Singer. On January 22 Singer reported on a study that showed that women who had implants had a higher risk of infection than women who had reconstruction using their own tissues. See "Study Says Implants Double Risk of Infection in Breast Reconstruction" in the *Times* or the original report in the *Archives of Surgery*, Vol. 143, No. 1, January 2008, by Margaret A. Olsen, Sorawuth Chu-Ongsakul, Keith E. Brandt, Jill R. Dietz, Jennie Mayfield, and Victoria J. Fraser, which you should look up just to see the rationale for the study: "Hospital-Associated Costs Due to Surgical Site Infection after Breast Surgery." Roni Caryn Rabin reported in the June 20, 2018, *Times* on a recent *JAMA Surgery* study by Dr. Edwin Wilkins that showed "One in three develop a postoperative complication over the next two years, and one in five requires more surgery. In 5 percent of cases, reconstruction fails." Why do articles like this make my heart sing? Am I not empathetic? I think I'm still insecure about my non-reconstructed breast and I like finding reasons that bolster my decision. Which I could reverse whenever I want.

February 20: *Blut und Boden* was the Nazi philosophy of Blood and Soil: the people of German blood belonged to the land and had a right to it.

April 22: In case you're wondering about the consequences of hope and "negativity" among cancer patients, see "Psychotherapy and Survival in Cancer: The Conflict Between Hope and Evidence" by James C. Coyne, Michael Stefanek, and Steven C. Palmer in the American Psychological Association's *Psychological Bulletin*, Vol. 133, No. 3, published in the summer of 2007. The authors criticize a famous 1989 study by Stanford University psychiatrist David Spiegel showing that women who attended support groups for breast cancer had a higher survival rate than those who didn't. My friend Garry Cooper, an articulate advocate of pessimism, discusses the article in the Clinician's Digest section of the *Psychotherapy Networker*, May/June 2008. He also reports on a study that found that placebos worked as well as antidepressants. Not on this Cancer Bitch.

"Hope and cancer" by psychologist David B. Feldman and oncologist Bejamin W. Corn, is an article that reviews thirty-three other studies and concludes that hope improves quality of life, "social support, and spiritual and existential well-being," and helps keep distress and depression at bay. That is common sense. However, oncologists were afraid to talk about advance care planning, because they feared it would "take away hope." I can see that. We want you to be hopeful, but please write down what your children should do when you're on your death bed. This was in *Current Opinion in Psychology Volume 49*, February 2023.

But people love hope. Why else would they keep going around quoting Anne Frank on it? She was hopeful when she was hiding in the Secret Annex in Amsterdam. I wager that she wasn't so hopeful when she was dying of typhus in Bergen-Belsen. Is it a disrespect to her death to be uplifted by her bouts of optimism? The people responsible for her death were not "good at heart." That diary entry continues: "I hear the ever approaching thunder, which will destroy us too…"

June 1: On the carcinogenic properties of plastics disposal, I originally consulted *State of the Evidence 2008: The Connection between Breast Cancer and the Environment*, edited by Janet Gray, Ph.D. The most recent update of the report I could find is from 2017. See the citation on April 9 or find on Breast Cancer Prevention Partners' site: https://www.bcpp.org/resource/state-evidence-2017. BCPP's motto is "Exposing the cause is the cure."

Post-Postscript: May 27, 2024: Lorde for some reason mistakenly called Moshe Dayan (1915-81) the prime minister of Israel. He was well known, unmistakable with that trademark eyepatch, so maybe he seemed to hold a higher office than he did. He served as defense minister and foreign minister. She spelled his first name *Moishe*, a Yiddishy version. That seems more Jewish, more *haimish*, homey, to me.

Acknowledgments:

First, I want to thank everyone who reached out after my diagnosis, whether by sending a card or plant or by asking how I was feeling. I'm grateful to my husband Linc Cohen for being the consummate cancer-spouse who always said and did the right thing (regarding my cancer, at least) and documented my hair loss and gain. My mother and sister provided support in person and via phone and e-mail and I knew they were always available. I'm grateful to my friends for escorting me to chemo, decorating my head, making dinner, bearing gifts and spending time with me. To wit:

Associate escort and compañera: Evelyn Wisenberg

Chief head-decorator, manuscript reader, chemo escort: Sharon Solwitz

Associate head-decorater, manuscript reader, chemo escort: Garnett Kilberg Cohen

Cameo head-decorator and long-distance supporter: Jennifer Berman

Manuscript reader and bearer of gifts: Maggie Kast

Traveling chemo escorts and supporters: Sylvienne Duryea, Dan Howell, Roz Fink

Manuscript consultant, hospital escort and accomplice: Peggy Shinner

Manuscript consultant and bearer of gifts: Tsivia Cohen

Manuscript consultant: Barry Silesky

Official Cancer Bitch yogi: Joyce Lanton

Official Cancer Bitch Chicago coffee houses: Emerald City Coffee (RIP; Café Avanti, (RIP); Bourgeois Pig Café, 738 W. Fullerton Pkwy., Letizia's Natural Bakery, 2144 W. Division St.; Dollop Coffee Co., 4181 N. Clarendon Ave.; 2024 coffee houses include Osmium Coffee Bar, 1117 W. Belmont; Kopi Café, 5317 N. Clark

The people at Chicago Public Radio who put the Cancer Bitch nineteen-part series on the program Eight Forty-Eight: Senior producer and wise editor Aurora Aguilar, producer and voice coach extraordinaire Ashley Gross, host Steve Edwards, interim host Gabriel Spitzer

Bearers of gifts, tangible and intangible: Robin Rich, Dorreen and Bill Carey, Jack Weinberg and Valerie Denney, Tara Ison, Chuck Burack, Kathy Price Westmoreland, Cecily Watson Burleson, Jan Levit-Silver, Bruce Campbell, Kathy Friedman, Cory Fosco, Rick Wirick, Rosellen Brown and Marv Hoffman, Anand and Maureen Aidasani, Jocelyn Hoffman and Jason Ewing, Phil Berger, Steve Jordan, Reg Gibbons, Miles Harvey, Barbara Rose, Wendy and Tom Kincaid, Natalia Rachel Singer, Julia Klein, Paula Barvin, Don Wiener, Jodi Cohen, Simone Muench, Beth Snyder, Steve Stabile and Andy Defuniak, Ladette Randolph, Ann Tyler, Barbara Ghoshal, Fred Cohen, Steve Marsden and Rebecca Rosenbaum, Tom Montgomery-Fate, Andy Cassel and C.J. Smith, Margie Smith Maidman and Janet, Paula and Irving Pozmantier

Health-care providers: Lora DeQuerido, Deborah Garcia Montero, Nora Hansen, Anaadriana Zakarija, Gina Uthe, Katie Marquardt, Merlita Cruzat-Blanco, Sandra Sheinin, James Urkov, Marc Feder, XueHua Feng, the phriendly phlebotomists at Fancy Hospital

Chief organizer, Cancer Bitch Headquarters: Jessica Rosenberg

My winter quarter '07 creative nonfiction class, which bore with me: Magdalen Dale, Bora Un, Elizabeth Winkowski, Amanda Mitchell Gebhardt, Allison Buell, Jenny McGrath, Laura Svendsen

Loyal blog readers: Stephanie Friedman, Cary Nathenson, Garry Cooper, Claudia Springer, Sam Harnish, Judith Bernstein, Lois Barr, Tim Chapman (who convinced me to go with Bitch instead of Babe), Anita Cohen, Baba Young, Vera Szabo, Dinah Wisenberg Brin, Josh Cohen

Friends and associates in the blogosphere and media: Jenni Prokopy at ChronicBabe.com, Paula Kamen, Mary Schmich, The

Fifty Foot Blogger, http://brys.wordpress.com, Jessica Wakeman at the *Huffington Post* blog, Brian Hieggelke at *NewCity Chicago*, ChemoChicks.com, EarthHenna.com, Bellaire74.com, Stephanie G'Schwind at the *Colorado Review*, Wendy, Summer Winter at the Pinch

For the first edition of the book: University of Iowa Press past and present staff Joe Parsons, Charlotte Wright, Holly Carver, James McCoy, Allison Thomas Means

For this first paperback edition: Jerry Brennan at Tortoise Books, for giving the book new life

If I forgot anyone, please forgive me. I want to list the places I've spoken and read my work, so that you will invite me to your institution, but that seems too much like marketing. You can get that information elsewhere. Like SLWisenberg.com, and adventures ofcancerbitch.com

I'm on socials as SL Wisenberg and Sandi Wisenberg, and on Facebook at Friends of Cancer Bitch

About the Author

S.L. Wisenberg is the author of *The Wandering Womb: Essays in Search of Home*, winner of the Juniper Prize in nonfiction, published by the University of Massachusetts Press in 2023. She's also the author of a short-story collection, *The Sweetheart Is In*; an essay collection, *Holocaust Girls: History, Memory, & Other Obsessions*. She is a fourth-generation Texan who lives in Chicago, where she is executive editor of *Another Chicago Magazine*. She's been awarded a Pushcart Prize and fellowships from the Illinois Arts Council, Fine Arts Work Center in Provincetown, National Endowment for the Humanities, and the city of Chicago. The first edition of *The Adventures of Cancer Bitch* was published by the University of Iowa Press. She's presented her work at many universities and cancer centers. Find her at SLwisenberg.com

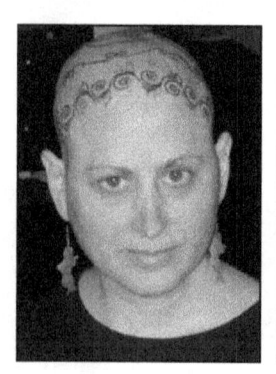

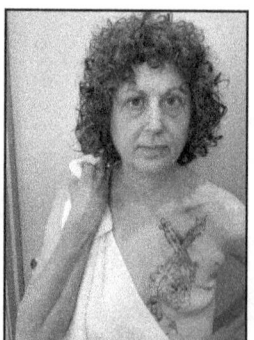

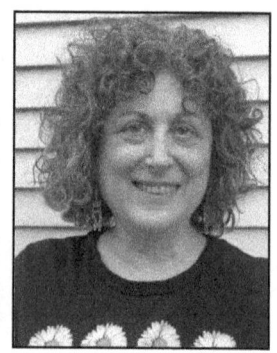

About Tortoise Books

Slow and steady wins in the end, even in publishing. Tortoise Books is dedicated to finding and promoting quality authors who haven't yet found a niche in the marketplace—writers producing memorable and engaging works that will stand the test of time.

Learn more at www.tortoisebooks.com or follow us on Twitter/X (assuming the website still exists when you're reading this) @TortoiseBooks.